Essentials of Ophthalmology

For Medical School and Beyond

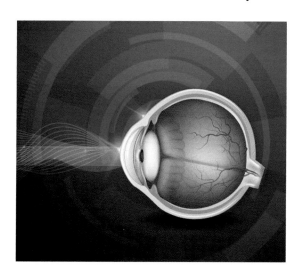

Essentials of Ophthalmology

For Medical School and Beyond

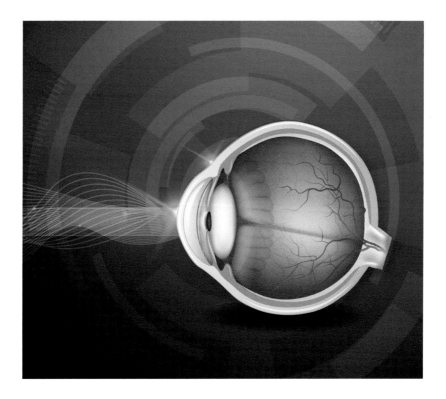

Editors

Ray Manotosh
Victor Koh

National University Hospital, Singapore

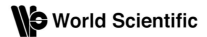

World Scientific

NEW JERSEY · LONDON · SINGAPORE · BEIJING · SHANGHAI · HONG KONG · TAIPEI · CHENNAI · TOKYO

Published by

World Scientific Publishing Co. Pte. Ltd.

5 Toh Tuck Link, Singapore 596224

USA office: 27 Warren Street, Suite 401-402, Hackensack, NJ 07601

UK office: 57 Shelton Street, Covent Garden, London WC2H 9HE

Library of Congress Cataloging-in-Publication Data

Names: Manotosh, Ray, editor. | Koh, Victor, editor.

Title: Essentials of ophthalmology : for medical school and beyond / editors, Ray Manotosh, Victor Koh.

Other titles: Essentials of ophthalmology (Manotosh)

Description: New Jersey : World Scientific, 2018. | Includes bibliographical references.

Identifiers: LCCN 2018038900| ISBN 9789813275591 (hardcover : alk. paper) |
    ISBN 9813275596 (hardcover : alk. paper)

Subjects: | MESH: Eye Diseases--therapy | Eye--anatomy & histology

Classification: LCC RE46 | NLM WW 166 | DDC 617.7--dc23

LC record available at https://lccn.loc.gov/2018038900

British Library Cataloguing-in-Publication Data

A catalogue record for this book is available from the British Library.

For any available supplementary material, please visit
https://www.worldscientific.com/worldscibooks/10.1142/11137#t=suppl

Printed in Singapore by Mainland Press Pte Ltd.

FOREWORD

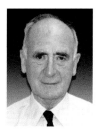

James F. (Barry) Cullen, MD, FRCS, FRCSEd. Formerly visiting
Professor and Consultant Neuro-Ophthalmologist
National University Hospital, Singapore

Essentials of Ophthalmology—for Medical School and Beyond continues the
tradition in the Department of Ophthalmology, National University of
Singapore (NUS) of providing a locally authored textbook, which was
first established in 1979 by the late Professor Arthur Lim (1934–2014)
with the *Colour Atlas of Ophthalmology*. Teaching and training of local and
overseas ophthalmologists was consolidated in Singapore in 1986 with the
establishment of the University Department of Ophthalmology at Kent
Ridge with Professor Lim as its first head and professor.

For most medical practitioners not in the specialty, ophthalmology
may appear as a collection of unpronounceable terms, rare syndromes,
unusual acronyms and mysterious conditions whereas in fact, it is an
entirely logical specialty where everything is visible to the examiner and
a diagnosis easily determined if an ordered approach to history taking
and examination is undertaken as pointed out in this book.

With the invention of the ophthalmoscope in 1850 by von Helmholtz, a
whole new world became visible! With modern photographic and imaging
techniques as depicted through the pages of this book, ophthalmology has
become a precise diagnostic discipline for both ophthalmic and medical
conditions.

Furthermore, due to the differences in disease patterns between South
East Asian and Caucasian populations, it is important that a locally
orientated text is available for medical students, ophthalmology trainees,
emergency medicine physicians, etc. who will all find this book of assistance
in their daily activities and is highly recommended to them all.

PREFACE

With so many Ophthalmology textbooks available, one wonders if there is sufficient motive to write yet another. Of course, there is the value of putting the necessary emphasis on conditions that are more common and more important locally. In the Singapore ophthalmology context, myopia, angle closure and polypoidal choroidal vasculopathy spring to mind. Furthermore, there are differences in healthcare provision and medical education systems. We have been told that we are fortunate to still have a dedicated two-week rotation in Ophthalmology. And perhaps this is still pertinent for Singapore as primary eye care that relies on other eye care professionals such as optometrists remains comparatively less developed and so the burden of primary eye care falls largely on family physicians.

The other important change that has occurred in the last decade is the push to have more of the didactic component of teaching move to Internet-based resources so that there is more time for patient-based learning and interactive learning. As we started preparing material for online learning, it seemed to make sense to us to simultaneously prepare a textbook for students as an additional resource for learning.

A textbook is, of course, no small undertaking, particularly where multiple authors are involved. Our tireless editors, Ray and Victor with the able assistance of Ives Yap, patiently planned, cajoled and pushed us all to get this tome written.

Perhaps more than anything else, this book is a labour of love for the Department of Ophthalmology of the National University Hospital and National University of Singapore. We wanted it to be a demonstration of our love for teaching and commitment to the education of medical students, residents and other eye care professionals. This commitment is a legacy left to us by our teachers and one that we hope to pass on to our students and all readers of this book.

Clement Tan Woon Teck, MBBS, MMed (Ophth), FRCSEd, FAMS
Head & Senior Consultant
Department of Ophthalmology
National University Hospital

ACKNOWLEDGEMENTS

We sincerely thank National University Health System, Singapore, for giving us this opportunity to write this text book as a part of the prestigious NUHS Text Book series.

Special thanks to all the contributors who dedicated their valuable time to write this book, without whom this work would not have been possible.

We would wish to thank Associate Professor Nga Min En and Dr Anita Lim for guiding us with constructive advice. We thank Ms Carolina Young and Vanessa Woo from Medical Affairs- Education, in facilitating the progress to publication.

We would like to acknowledge the continuous encouragement that we received from our Head of Department, Associate Professor Clement Tan, who also contributed immensely to this book. We are especially grateful to Prof Barry Cullen who kindly agreed to write the Foreword for this book.

Last but not the least, no words can express our gratitude to Ms Ives Yap, our Undergraduate Program Coordinator who worked tirelessly to make this publication possible.

ABOUT THE EDITORS

Ray Manotosh

Ray Manotosh is currently a Senior Consultant in Ophthalmology at the National University Health System, Singapore. His field of specialisation is Cornea, External Eye Diseases, Contact Lens and Refractive Surgery. He is also Assistant Professor and Undergraduate Medical Education Director of Ophthalmology at the Yong Loo Lin School of Medicine, National University of Singapore. Concurrently he is involved in postgraduate residency program in the capacity of core faculty at National University Hospital, Singapore.

Dr. Ray completed his undergraduate training at the University of Calcutta, India. He completed basic surgical training in Ophthalmology at the prestigious All India Institute of Medical Sciences (AIIMS), New Delhi, the premier medical institute in India. He obtained his MD (Ophthalmology) in 1997. Subsequently he underwent advanced surgical training in the field of cornea and external diseases at AIIMS. He is also a Fellow in Ophthalmology at the Royal College of Surgeons of Edinburgh (UK) since 1998. After completing the advanced surgical training, he joined National University Hospital, Singapore in 2002. In 2006, Dr. Ray attained the NHG Excellence Award for teaching. He has published in many peer-reviewed journals as well as contributed many text book chapters.

Dr. Ray enjoys spending time with his family and spends his leisure hours in painting, writing and jogging.

Victor Koh

Victor Koh is a Consultant Ophthalmologist with a special interest in the management of glaucoma and cataracts. He graduated from NUS Yong Loo Lin School of Medicine in 2007 and obtained specialist accreditation in 2016. His research interests centres around Medtech and he holds several grants/patents to develop novel devices/algorithms to improve ophthalmic care in the community. He modeled his practice after his inspiring teachers who included A/Prof. Paul Chew, A/Prof. Clement Tan, Dr. Loon Seng Chee, Prof. Aung Tin and Dr. Aliza Jap. Victor would like to give special thanks to his wife and two boys who have been his pillar of support throughout most parts of his training years.

LIST OF CONTRIBUTORS

Anna Marie Tan Wee Tien, MBBS, MMed (Ophth), MRCSEd
Senior Consultant & Residency Program Director
Head, Division of Cornea & Refractive Surgery

Clement Tan Woon Teck, MBBS, MMed (Ophth), FRCSEd , FAMS
Head & Senior Consultant
Department of Ophthalmology
National University Hospital
Head, Division of Neuro-Ophthalmology

Chai Hui Chen Charmaine, MBBS, MMed (Ophth), FAMS
Consultant
Division of Cornea & Refractive Surgery

Chan Hwei Wuen, MBBS, MMed (Ophth), FAMS, FRCOphth (UK)
Consultant
Division of Vitreo-retina & Electrophysiology

Chen Ziyou David, MBBS
Resident, Ophthalmology

Cheryl Ngo Shufen, MBBS, MMed (Ophth), FRCSEd (Ophth)
Consultant
Head, Division of Paediatric Ophthalmology

Danial Bohan, BSc (Hons), MSc
Senior Optometrist

Dawn Lim Ka-Ann, MBBS, MRCP (UK), MMed (Int.Med), MMed (Ophth), FAMS
Consultant
Division of Ocular inflammation & Glaucoma

Gangadhara Sundar, DO, FRCSEd, FAMS
Senior Consultant
Head, Division of Orbit & Oculofacial surgery

George Thomas Naveen, MBBS, MMed (Ophth)
Associate Consultant, Ophthalmology

Goh Miao Jin, MBBS
Former Resident of Ophthalmology

Jeyabal Preethi, MBBS
Medical Officer, Ophthalmology

Koh Teck Chang Victor, MBBS, MMed(Ophth), MRCSEd, FAMS
Consultant
Division of Glaucoma

Lam Sing Harn Janice, MBBS, MMed (Ophth)
Associate Consultant
Division of Paediatric Ophthalmology

Lim Xiaohong Blanche, MBBS, MMed (Ophth)
Senior Resident, Ophthalmology

Lin Hui'en Hazel Anne, MBBS, MMed (Ophth), FAMS
Associate Consultant
Division of Neuro-ophthalmology

Marcus Tan Chun Jin, MBBS, MMed (Ophth)
Senior Resident, Ophthalmology

Paul Zhao Song Bo, MBBS, MMed (Ophth), FRCSEd (Ophth)
Consultant
Division of Vitreo-retina

Ray Manotosh, MBBS, MD (AIIMS), FRCSEd
Senior Consultant & Undergraduate Program Director
Division of Cornea & Refractive Surgery

Shantha Amrith, MD (Ophth), AIMS, DO, FRCS(Ed), FRCOphth, FAMS
Senior Consultant
Division of Orbit & Oculofacial surgery

Stephanie Ming Young, MBBS, MMed (Ophth), FRCOphth, FAMS
Consultant
Division of Orbit & Oculofacial surgery

Teoh Chin Sheng, MD
Resident, Ophthalmology

Yuen Yew Sen, MBBS, MMed (Ophth), FAMS
Associate Consultant
Division of Vitreo-retina & Ocular inflammation

CONTENTS

BASIC ANATOMY OF THE EYE, ADNEXA AND VISUAL PATHWAYS

1.1 Basic Anatomy

Learning Objectives
Understand the basic anatomical structures of the globe.

The external structure of the globe comprises the sclera (outer most layer), uveal tissue (middle layer) and retina (innermost layer). Refer to Fig. 1.1.

Sclera

- Strong and dense coat protecting the intraocular contents
- Anterior 1/6th — transparent cornea, posterior 5/6th opaque sclera. Junction is called limbus

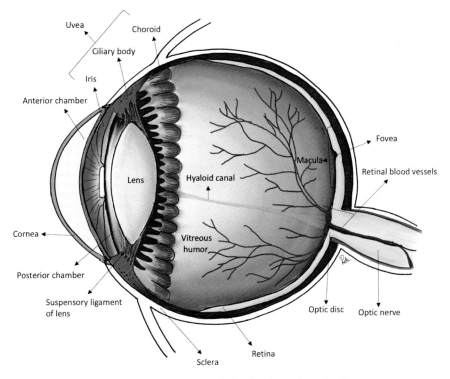

Fig. 1.1. Coronal section of the eyeball showing the various structures.

- Thickness:
  - Thickest posteriorly (1 mm) and gradually becomes thinner upon tracing anteriorly
  - Thinnest at the level of insertion of extraocular muscles
- Lamina cribrosa: sieve-like part of sclera through which optic nerves exits the globe

Uveal tissue

- Supplies nutrition to various structures of the eyeball
- From anterior to posterior, it consists of iris, ciliary body and choroid
- Functions:
  - Iris: iris colour varies among different individuals depending on the amount of melanin. Controls amount of light entering the eye
  - Ciliary body: aqueous humour production, accommodation
  - Choroid: supplies oxygen and nutrition to outer layers of retina

Retina

- See the sections below for more details

Take home messages

The cornea and sclera forms the outermost wall of the globe and forms a protective cover over the intraocular structures.

1.2 Cornea

Learning Objectives

Understand the components and functions of the different layers of the cornea.

The cornea is the transparent outermost covering of the eye and is the most important refractive medium of the eye (Fig. 1.2 and Fig. 1.3).

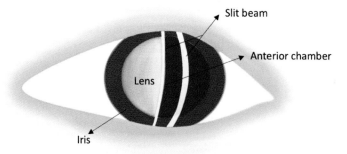

Fig. 1.2. Illustration of slit-lamp beam image of the anterior segment. The first broad slit beam corresponds to the cornea and the second narrow beam corresponds to the anterior surface of the lens.

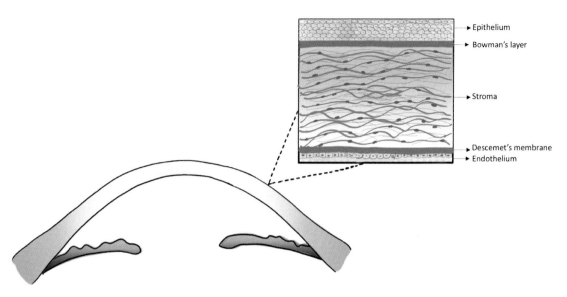

Fig. 1.3. Cross-section of the cornea and the 5 layers.

The 5 layers of the cornea are composed of:

Epithelium

- 5 layers of cells and 50-60 microns thick
- Approximately 7 days for complete turnover of corneal surface epithelium
- Production of new cells occurs at the limbus and grows centripetally from the periphery towards the centre
- Nerve endings of sensory nerve fibres run between the epithelial cells

Bowman's Layer

- Acellular layer
- 8–12 microns thick

Stroma

- Forms 90% of corneal thickness
- Multiple lamellae of compact collagen fibrils
- Uniform spacing of collagen fibrils maintain the transparency

Descemet's Membrane

- Basement membrane of the endothelium
- 10 microns thick

Endothelium

- Single layer of flattened cells
- Important in the transport of fluid, keeping the cornea dehydrated and transparent
- Does not regenerate
- Physiological rate of loss of cells with age

Nerve Supply of the Cornea

- From the ophthalmic division of the trigeminal nerve (mainly through the long ciliary nerves)
- Forms the annular plexus at the limbus
- Branches pass radially into the stroma
- Branches unite to form subepithelial plexus
- Terminal branches pass the bowman membrane and form the intraepithelial plexus

Important Features of the Cornea

Avascular

- Receives its nutrients from diffusion from the aqueous humour and dissolved oxygen from the tear film

No Lymphatic Drainage

- Avascularity and the absence of immune cells in the cornea makes it an immune-privileged site for grafting

Nerve Plexus

- Naked nerve endings that run in the epithelium result in intense pain in the presence of a corneal abrasion

Limbal Stem Cells

- Found at the limbus and are important for regeneration of new epithelial cells

Endothelial Pump

- Corneal oedema occurs due to fluid entering the stromal leading to a loss of the regularity of the stromal collagen fibrils
- This can occur due to insufficient endothelial cells or from dysfunction of the cells (e.g trauma or acute rise in intraocular pressure)

Take home messages
- There are 5 distinct layers of the cornea and each plays an important role in the overall function of the cornea.
- The cornea endothelium does not regenerate.

1.3 Anterior Chamber Angle

Learning Objectives
- The components and position of each part of the anterior chamber angle from a gonioscopic view.
- Understand the aqueous outflow dynamics and pathways.

The angle of the anterior chamber is made up of the Schwalbe's line, anterior and posterior trabecular meshwork, scleral spur and ciliary body. These structures are involved in the

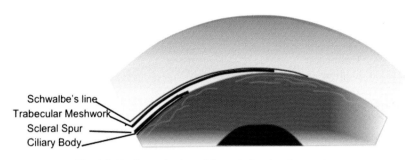

Schwalbe's line
Trabecular Meshwork
Scleral Spur
Ciliary Body

Fig. 1.4. Gonioscopic view of the anterior chamber angle.

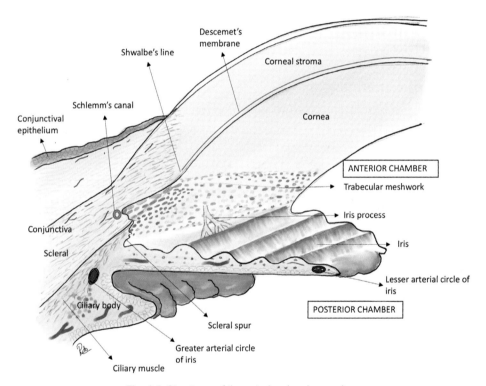

Fig. 1.5. Structures of the anterior chamber angle.

production and drainage of aqueous humour of the eye and maintenance of the intraocular pressure (Fig. 1.4 and Fig. 1.5).

The anterior segment is made up of the cornea, anterior chamber, iris, lens, ciliary body and the anterior part of the sclera. The anterior chamber is bound anteriorly by the cornea and posteriorly by the iris and pupil, while the posterior chamber is bound anteriorly by the iris and posteriorly by the ciliary body and lens. Aqueous humour fills both the anterior and posterior chamber.

Flow of Aqueous Humour

- Produced at the ciliary body (Fig. 1.6)
- Flows anterior to the lens and through the pupil

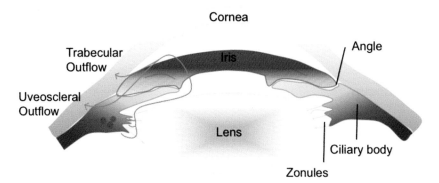

Fig. 1.6. Dynamics of the aqueous humour.

- 90% drain through the trabecular meshwork into the Schlemm's canal
- 10% drain via the uveo-scleral pathway

Function of Aqueous Humour

- Maintenance of intraocular pressure and structural form of the globe
- Provide nutrition to surrounding tissues such as the posterior cornea, trabecular meshwork and lens
- For its refractive index

Take home messages

- The posterior trabecular meshwork is an important landmark in the gonioscopic view due to its function in aqueous outflow.
- Aqueous outflow from the eye is mainly from the trabecular meshwork and uveo-scleral pathway.

1.4 Vitreous

Learning Objectives

Understand the composition and function of the vitreous gel.

- Viscous, gel — like fluid that is composed of 99 % water and mainly type II and some type IX collagen fibres, mucopolysaccharides and hyaluronic acid
- Volume 4 mL
- Functions:
  - Mechanical stabilisation of volume of globe
  - Shock absorption
  - Nutrition supply to lens and retina
- As we age, syneresis (liquefaction) occurs

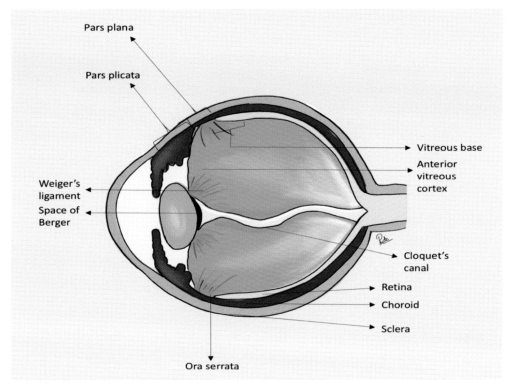

Fig.1.7. Vitreous anatomy and the vitreoretinal junctions.

Vitreous Base

- Portion of vitreous that is attached to peripheral retina and pars plana
- It is 6 mm wide (straddling the ora serrata — 2 mm anterior and 4 mm posterior to it)
- The vitreous base in tightly adherent to the ora serrata

Vitreoretinal Junctions

- Firm attachment between vitreous and retina at level of foot plate of Muller's cells at internal limiting membrane.
- Locations of vitreoretinal junctions (Fig. 1.7):
  - Vitreous base — strongest
  - Margin of optic disc
  - Fovea
  - Back of lens
  - Areas of chorioretinal scars
  - Edges of lattice degeneration
- Blunt trauma may cause avulsion of vitreous base which may lead to tearing of the retina along its posterior border

- Posterior vitreous detachment is separation of cortical vitreous from the retina anywhere posterior to the vitreous base

> **Take home messages**
> • The vitreous is a clear media which acts as a shock absorbent for the eye.
> • There are firm adhesions between the vitreous and the retina which might result in retinal tears or detachment.

1.5 Retina

> **Learning Objectives**
> • Identify the different layers of the retina and their boundaries.
> • Understand the functions of the retina and how the different components contribute to vision.

- Retina forms the inner nervous coat of the eyeball
  - It extends from the optic disc posteriorly to the ora serrata anteriorly
- Retina is divided into posterior pole and peripheral retina by the equator
  - Equator is an imaginary circle drawn at the level of exit of the 4 vortex veins
- Optic disc
  - Circular area of approximately 1500 μm in diameter
  - Nerve fibres exit the retina through the lamina cribrosa to run into the optic nerve
  - Optic cup is a physiological depression seen in the disc. The central retinal artery and vein emerge through the centre of this cup
- Macula lutea
  - 5500 μm area located at the posterior pole temporal to the optic disc (Fig. 1.8)
  - Fovea centralis is the central depressed part of macula, about 1500 μm in diameter
  - Foveola is the central shiny pit, about 350 μm in diameter, located 2 disc diameter temporal to the optic disc and 1 mm below the horizontal meridian
  - Foveal avascular zone comprises the foveola and some area surrounding it (total of 800 μm in diameter) that is devoid of any retinal capillaries
- Ora serrata
  - Serrated peripheral margin forming the anterior boundary of retina
  - Retina is attached firmly to vitreous and choroid
  - Pars plana extends anteriorly from the ora serrata

Layers of Retina

Based on light microscopy, the retina is made up of 10 layers from outward to inwards (Fig. 1.9)

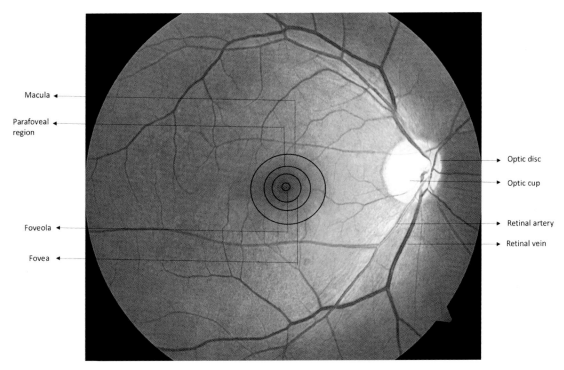

Fig.1.8. Fundus photograph showing the posterior pole and its important landmarks.

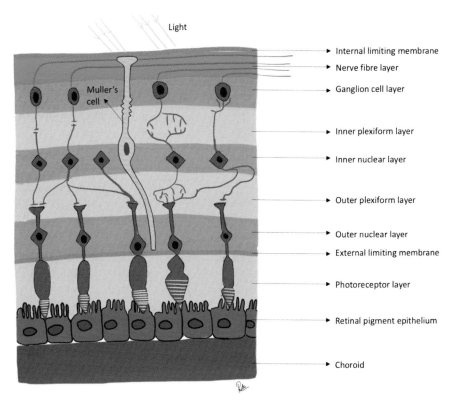

Fig. 1.9. Layers of the retina demonstrating various neuronal connections.

Pigment Epithelium

- Outermost layer consisting of single layer of cells containing pigment
- Firmly adherent to underlying basal lamina (Bruch's membrane) of choroid
- Functions:
  - Absorptions of light, blood retinal barrier, visual pigment regeneration and synthesis, removal of debris from photoreceptors by phagocytic action

Photoreceptor Layer

- Layer of rods and cones (photoreceptors) arranged in a palisade manner
- Human eye consists of about 120 million rods and 6.5 million cones
- Functions:
  - Rods—night (scotopic) vision and peripheral vision
  - Cones—day light (photopic) vision and colour vision
- Rods and cones are the end-organs of vision that transform light energy into visual (nerve) impulse

External Limiting Membrane

- Junction between cell membrane of photoreceptors and Muller's cells
- The processes of rods and cones pass through this fenestrated membrane
- Functions:
  - Selective barrier for nutrients
  - Stabilisation of transducing portion of photoreceptors

Outer Nuclear Layer

- Nuclei of rods and cones

Outer Plexiform Layer

- Connections of rod spherules and cone pedicle with dendrites of bipolar and horizontal cells
- Functions:
  - Transmission and amplification of electric potential
  - Functional barrier to diffusion of fluids and metabolites
- Clinical significance: Hard exudates, dot and blot haemorrhges are found in this layer

Inner Nuclear Layer

- Bipolar, horizontal and amacrine cell bodies
- Function: Numerous cells and extensive cellular connections of INL is essential for transduction and amplification of light signals
- Bipolar cells — first order neurons. Relay information from photoreceptors to horizontal, amacrine and ganglion cells
- Horizontal cells — modulates and transform visual information received from photoreceptors
- Amacrine cells — modulates the electrical information reaching the ganglion cells

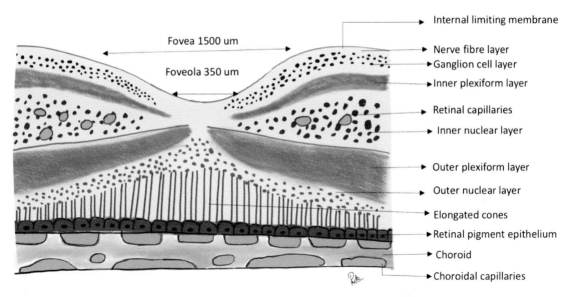

Fig. 1.10. Cross-section at the fovea. Note the difference in architecture of the layers at the fovea compared to rest of the retina.

Inner Plexiform Layer

- Connections of axons of bipolar cells with dendrites of ganglion cells and processes of amacrine cells

Ganglion Cell Layer

- Cell bodies of ganglion cells. (second order neurons)
- Function: Transmission of signals from bipolar cells to lateral geniculate body

Nerve Fibre Layer

- Axons of ganglion cells
- Usually unmyelinated within the retina
- Clinical significance: Cotton wool spots and flame shaped haemorrhages are found in this layer

Internal Limiting Membrane

- Innermost layer of retina separating it from the vitreous
- Basement membrane formed by union of terminal expansions of Muller's cells

Structure of Fovea Centralis (Fig. 1.10)

- Fovea: 1500 µm central depression of inner retinal surface within the macula
- Corresponds to FAZ (foveal avascular zone)
- No rods. Cones are tightly packed and other layers of retina are thin
- Contains taller RPE cells and xanthophyll pigments
- Foveola: 350 µm avascular central area of fovea. Absence of ganglion cells and other nucleated cells.

Why is fovea dark?

RPE cells at the fovea are taller, thinner and contain more pigment granules, thereby giving a dark color to this area as compared to rest of the retina.

Blood Supply of the Retina

- The central retinal artery is a branch of ophthalmic artery. It is an end artery that enters the optic nerve nearly 1 cm behind the globe. After emerging from centre of the optic cup, they divide into 4 branches (supero-nasal, supero-temporal, infero-nasal and infero-temporal)
- Retinal veins follow the pattern of arteries. Drains into cavernous sinus either directly or via the superior ophthalmic vein
- Inner 6 layers of retina are supplied by the central retinal artery
- Outer 4 layers are supplied by choroidal vessels

Take home messages

- There are 10 layers of the retina and each layer plays a different function.
- Macula is further subdivided into 3 zones.
- The photoreceptors comprise of cones and rods and they are distributed differently in the retina.
- There is dual blood supply to the retinal layers.

1.6 Eyelid

Learning Objectives

- Understand the topographical and cross-sectional anatomy of the eyelid - blood and nerve supply.
- Learn the function of the eyelid.

Lamellae of Upper Eyelid (Fig. 1.11 and Fig. 1.12)

Anterior: skin, orbicularis
Posterior: tarsus, levator aponeurosis, Muller's muscle, palpebral conjunctiva

The following are the structures found in eyelids from superficial to deep:

Skin

- Thinnest in the body

Double eyelids

Attachment of fibres of the levator palpebrae superioris muscle to the upper eyelid skin creates eyelid crease. Nearly half of Asians have upper lids with a low but defined upper lid crease, which segments the eyelid into 2 visible parts called "double eyelids."

Subcutaneous Areolar Tissue

- Very loose and hence readily distended by oedema or blood
- No fat

Striated Muscle Layer

- Orbicularis oculi muscle
  - Comprises 3 parts — orbital, palpebral (pretarsal and preseptal parts) and lacrimal.

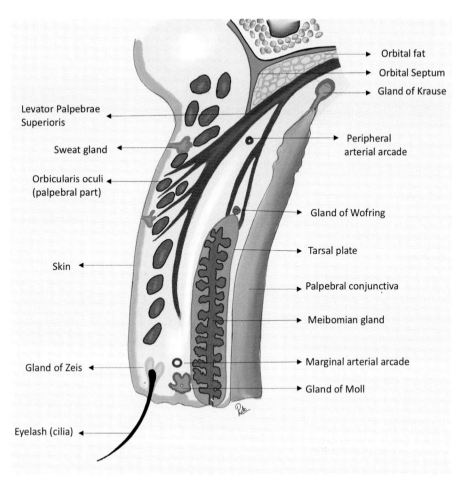

Fig. 1.11. Anatomy of the upper eyelid.

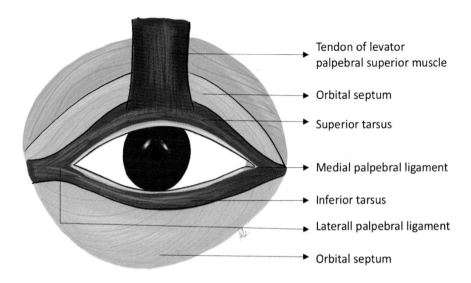

Fig. 1.12. Anatomy of the fibrous layer of eyelid showing tarsal plates and orbital septum.

- Function: closure of eyelids, main protractor of eyelid and acts as lacrimal pump
- Nerve supply: zygomatic branch of facial nerve
- Levator palpebrae superioris (LPS)
  - Origin: apex of orbit
  - Insertion: (by 3 parts) skin of eyelid, tarsal plate anterior surface and conjunctiva of superior fornix
  - Function: elevates the upper eyelid
  - Nerve supply: oculomotor nerve

Fibrous Layer

- Forms the structural framework of eyelids and consists of tarsal plate centrally and orbital septum peripherally
- Tarsal plate
  - Dense connective tissue layer
  - The upper and lower tarsal plates are connected at medial and lateral canthi
  - Medial and lateral palpebral ligaments provided attachment for tarsal plates with orbital margin
  - Meibomian glands and embedded in the tarsal plates
- Orbital septum
  - Forms a barrier between skin and orbit and eyelid; prevents spread of infection
  - Attachments: periosteum of orbital margin and tarsal plates

Non-striated Muscle Layer

- Palpebral muscle of Muller: lies deep to orbital septum
- Origin: upper lid — from fibres of LPS muscle; lower lid — prolongation of inferior rectus muscle
- Insertion: peripheral margin of tarsal plate
- Nerve supply: sympathetic fibres

Palpebral Conjunctiva

- Inner lining of eyelids
- 3 parts: marginal, tarsal and orbital

Landmarks on Eyelid Margins (Anterior to Posterior)

- Lash line: 2 to 3 rows of nearly 100 lashes in upper lid and 50 lashes in lower lid
- Gray line: junction of anterior and posterior lamellae. Vascular watershed area
- Meibomian gland orifices: nearly 30 in upper lid and 20 in lower lid

Eyelid laceration repair

For full thickness eyelid lacerations involving the lid margin, proper technique of repair involving suturing of conjunctiva, tarsal plate, gray line and skin sequentially is essential for restoring the structural integrity of eyelid.

Glands of Eyelids

Gland	Location	Features
Meibomian/tarsal	Within tarsus	Opens at lid margin Oily layer of tear film
Glands of Zeis	Near lid margin Associated with cilia	Opens into follicles of eyelashes Lubricates cilia
Glands of Moll	Near lid margin	Lubricates cilia
Accessory lacrimal glands: **Krause**	Superior fornix	Basal tear secretion (aqueous)
Wolfring	Just above tarsus	
Sweat gland		Electrolyte balance
Goblet cells	Conjunctiva Plica Caruncle	Mucin secretion Corneal wetting

Blood Supply

Arterial Supply

- Medial palpebral arteries (arising from ophthalmic artery) and lateral palpebral arteries (arising from lacrimal artery) form marginal arterial arcade
- Another arcade (superior arterial arcade) is present in upper lid. It lies near upper border of tarsus
- Anastomoses between facial artery (derived from external carotid) and palpebral arteries (derived from internal carotid) are present at medial and lateral aspect of eyelids

Venous Drainage

Arranged in 2 plexus:
- Pre-tarsal: opening into subcutaneous veins
- Post-tarsal: drains into ophthalmic vein

Lymphatics

Arranged in 2 sets:
- Pre- tarsal and post – tarsal
- Lateral ½ of lids drain into preauricular nodes and medial ½ drains into submandibular nodes

Nerve Supply

Motor

- Facial N — orbicularis muscle
- Oculomotor N — levator palpabrea superioris muscle
- Sympathetic fibers — Muller's muscle

Sensory

- Upper lid: branches of V1 of trigeminal nerve (lacrimal, supraorbital and supratrochlear)
- Lower lid: branches of V2 of trigeminal nerve (infratrochlear) along with branches of infraorbital (V1)

> **Take home messages**
> - The eyelid can be divided into the anterior and posterior lamellae.
> - There are 3 distinct landmarks on the eyelid margins which is relevant to eyelid laceration repair.

1.7 Orbit

> **Learning Objectives**
> - Understand the orbital wall boundaries and its bony parts.
> - Learn the relationship of the orbital walls with the blood and nerve supply that enters/exits the orbit.

The bony orbits are pear/pyramid shaped cavities sandwiched between the anterior cranial fossa and maxillary sinus; made up of 7 bones (Fig. 1.13).

Each orbit is about 30 ml in volume. One-fifth is occupied by the eyeball.

Floor

- Thin, triangular shaped
- Formed primarily by the orbital plate of maxilla with contributions from zygomatic and palatine bones
- Easily involved in orbital blow-out fractures and easily invaded by tumour of maxillary sinus

Lateral Wall

- Triangular; covers only posterior half of eyeball. Surgical approach to orbit via lateral orbitotomy is popular
- Formed by zygomatic bone anteriorly and greater wing of sphenoid posteriorly

Roof

- Formed by orbital plate of frontal bone and lesser wing of sphenoid
- Separates orbit from anterior cranial fossa

Medial Wall

- Medial wall of 2 orbits are parallel to each other
- Thinnest of orbital walls — frequently fractured
- Formed by maxilla, lacrimal, ethmoid and body of sphenoid bone

Orbital Apex

Posterior convergence of 4 orbital walls. Consists of the following 2 orifices (Fig. 1.14)

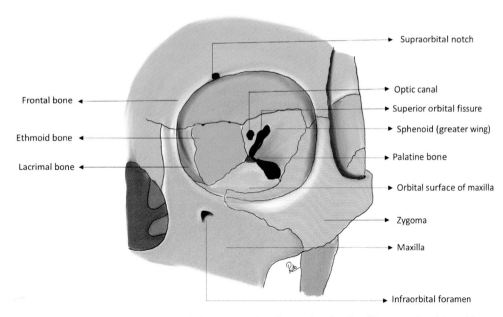

Fig. 1.13. Bony architecture of orbit. Note the various bones forming the different walls of the orbit.

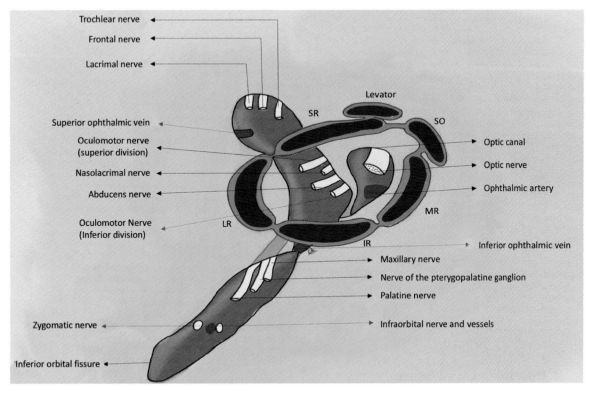

Fig. 1.14. Anatomy of superior and inferior orbital fissures. Note the various important structures traversing it.

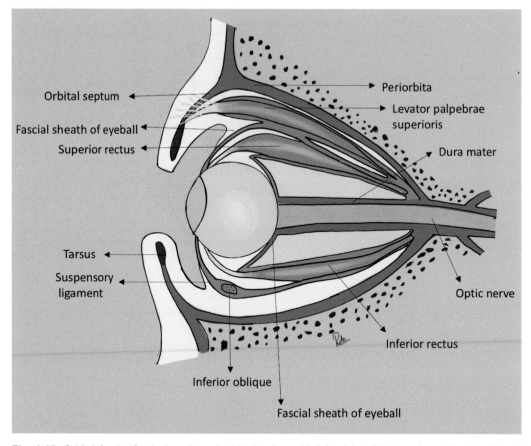

Fig. 1.15. Orbital fascia: Sagittal section of orbit showing orbital fascial architecture in relation to different structures.

Optic Canal

- Transmits optic nerve and ophthalmic artery

Superior Orbital Fissure

- Slit between cranium and orbit, lying between greater and lesser wings of sphenoid bones
- Lacrimal, frontal, trochlear nerve and superior ophthalmic vein pass through the superior orbital fissure above the tendinous ring
- Nasociliary, abducent and oculomotor nerve (superior and inferior divisions) pass inside the tendinous ring
- Inferior ophthalmic vein pass inferior to tendinous ring
- Inflammation of Superior Orbital Fissure or Orbital apex may result in multitude of signs like ophthalmoplegia and venous outflow obstruction

Inferior Orbital Fissure

- Slit between the greater wing of sphenoid and the maxilla
- Connects the orbit to the pterygopalatine and infraorbital fossae
- Continuous with the infraorbital canal
- Transmits branches of maxillary nerve, and an emissary vein connecting ophthalmic vein to pterygoid plexus

Orbital Fascia (Fig. 1.15)

- Thin connective tissue membrane lining various intraorbital structures
- Divided into fascia bulbi (Tenon's capsule) which envelopes the globe from limbus to optic nerve, muscular sheaths, intermuscular septa, membranous expansion of muscles and ligament of lockwood (thickened lower part in the form of a hammock or sling on which the globe sits)

Take home messages

- The orbit comprises 4 walls arranged in a pyramidal fashion and has 2 main orifices — optic canal and orbital fissure.
- The medial wall and floor of the orbit are thin and are prone to fractures in trauma.
- The orbital apex region has to accommodate multiple structures including the recti muscles, cranial nerves and large orbital vessels.

1.8 Lacrimal System

Learning Objectives
Understand the lacrimal drainage pathway of the eye.

Puncta (Fig. 1.16)

- 2 in number: upper and lower
- Located at the junction of the lash-bearing lateral 5/6th (pars cilia) and the medial non — ciliated 1/6th (pars lacrimalis), at the posterior edge of the lid margin about 6 mm from the medial canthus, lower slightly more temporal
- Slightly inverted against globe. Examined by everting the eyelid

Canaliculi

- 10 mm long (2 mm vertical segment [ampulla] and 8 mm horizontal portion parallel to lid margin)
- Combine to form single canaliculus in 90% of individuals
- Reflux from lacrimal sac to canaliculus is prevented by valve of Rosenmuller

Nasolacrimal Sac

- 10 – 12 mm long
- Lies between the anterior and posterior medial canthal tendon, lodged in the lacrimal fossa in between the anterior and posterior lacrimal crests
- Lies lateral to middle meatus of nose, separated by the lacrimal bone and frontal process of maxilla

Nasolacrimal Duct

- 12 – 18 mm long inferior continuation of the lacrimal sac

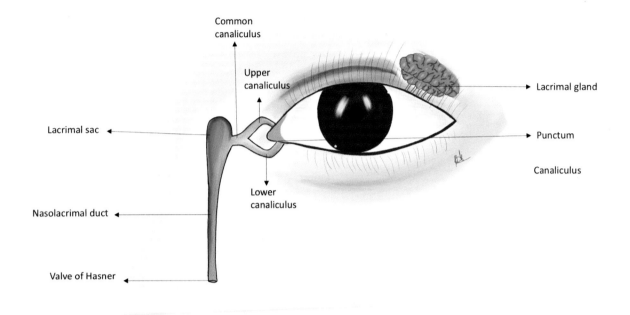

Fig. 1.16. Anatomy of the lacrimal system.

- Lies within the lacrimal canal formed by the maxillary and lacrimal bones, passing inferiorly, posteriorly and laterally
- Opens into the ipsilateral inferior meatus. Opening is covered by a partial fold of mucosa called valve of Hasner

Physiology

- Tears are secreted by main and accessory lacrimal gland, pass along the ocular surface and enter the upper and lower canaliculi by capillary action and suction
- When eyelids close, ampullae are compressed by pretarsal orbicularis oculi, horizontal canaliculi are shortened and compresses, puncta closed and moved medially, resisting reflux. Also, by the contraction of lacrimal part of orbicularis oculi, positive pressure created forcing tears down the nasolacrimal duct into the nose, mediated by connective tissue fibres around the sac
- When eyelids open, negative pressure created as the canaliculi and sac expand, drawing tears from the canaliculi into the sac

Take home messages
Tears drain from the puncta through the canaliculi and into the nasolacrimal sac/duct.

1.9 Visual Pathway

Learning Objectives
• Learn the visual pathway from the optic nerve up to the visual cortex.
• The relationship of the optic chiasm with the intracranial structures.
• Familiarise with reflex pupillary pathways.

Visual Pathway Comprises

Optic nerve, optic chiasm, optic tract, lateral geniculate body, optic radiations and visual cortex. Image from temporal part of visual field falls on nasal retina and vice versa for each eye.

Optic Nerve (Fig. 1.17)

• 47–50 mm in length.
• Distal continuation of nerve fiber layer of retina consisting of axon of ganglion cells
• Parts of optic nerve:
  ▪ Intraocular part (1 mm): Starts from optic disc and pierces the choroid and sclera (lamina cribrosa)
  ▪ Intraorbital part (25 mm- longest): Extends posteriorly until optic foramina, where it is surrounded by Annulus of Zinn (refer to Fig. 1.14). Optic nerve is myelinated posterior to lamina cribrosa. Central Retina Artery enters and central Retinal Vein exits the dural sheath here

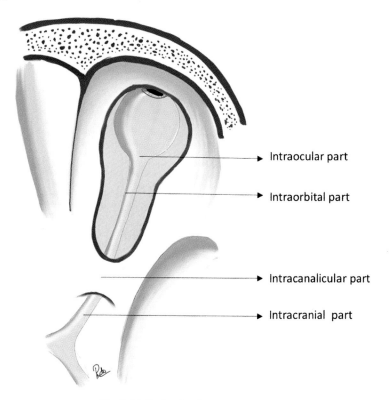

Intraocular part

Intraorbital part

Intracanalicular part

Intracranial part

Fig. 1.17. Parts of optic nerve.

- Intracanalicular part (5mm): Within the optic canal, the nerve is closely related to the ophthalmic artery which lies inferolaterally initially and later crossel obliquely over it to lie medially
- Intracranial part (10 mm): Travels upwards, backwards and medially to reach the optic chiasm

Optic Chiasm (Fig. 1.18)

- Location — Over the tuberculum and diaphragm sellae. Hence visual field defects are seen in patients with pituitary tumour having suprasellar extension
- Important relations
  - Superiorly: floor of 3rd ventricle, lamina terminalis and anterior communicating artery
  - Inferiorly: diaphragma sellae
  - Anteriorly: anterior cerebral artery
  - Posteriorly: tuber cinereum (base of pituitary stalk), mammillary bodies
  - Laterally: internal carotid artery and cavernous sinus
- Optic nerve fibres from nasal retina undergo decussation as the optic chiasm

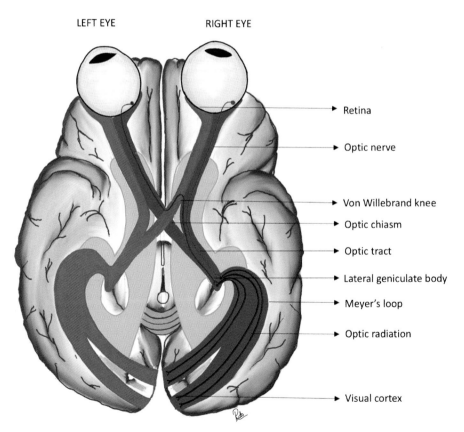

Fig. 1.18. Anatomy of the visual pathway.

Optic Tract

- Cylindrical bundle of nerve fibres extending outwards and backwards from posterolateral aspect of optic chiasm to lateral geniculate body (LGB)
- Contains fibres from temporal retina of ipsilateral eye and nasal retina of contralateral eye
- The pupillary reflex fibres pass on to pretectal nucleus bypassing the LGB

Lateral Geniculate Body

- Oval structures at termination of optic tract
- Consists of 6 layers of neurons
- Layers 2, 3 & 5 receive fibres from temporal retina of ipsilateral eye and layers 1, 4 & 6 receive fibres from nasal retina of opposite eye
- Second order neurons relay in LGB

Optic Radiations

- 3rd order neurons of visual pathway
- Extends from LGB to visual cortex passing forwards initially then laterally and then spreads out like a fan forming medullary optic lamina
- Superior fibres subserving inferior visual field traverse posteriorly through parietal lobe
- Inferior fibres subserving superior visual field sweep anteroinferiorly in Meyer's loop and traverse through temporal lobe

Visual Cortex

- Located at medial aspect of each occipital lobe, in the area above and below the calcarine fissure
- 2 divisions:
  - Primary visual cortex / visuosensory area: striate area 17
  - Secondary visual cortex / visuopsychic area: peristriate area 18 and parastriate area 19

Blood Supply of the Visual Pathway

Except the orbital part of optic nerve which is supplied by an axial system derived from the central retinal artery, the remainder of the visual pathway is supplied by pial network of vessels. The pial plexus gets contribution from different arteries at different levels of visual pathway as shown in Fig. 1.19

Blood Supply of the Optic Nerve (Fig. 1.20)

- Prelaminar portion: Centripetal branches from peripapillary choroidal vessels
- Lamina cribrosa: Short posterior ciliary arteries that form cicle of Zinn. No significant anastomoses with branches of the central retinal artery
- Retrolaminar: Mainly by centripetal branches from pial plexus and also from branches of central retinal artery

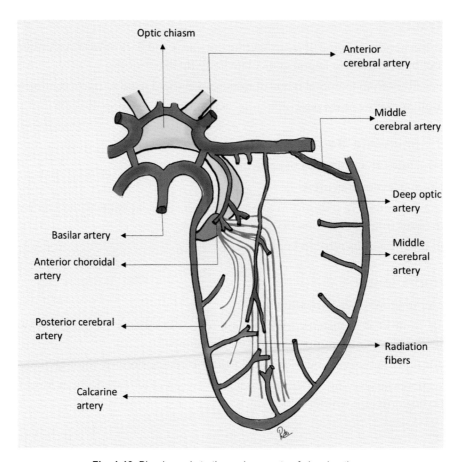

Fig. 1.19. Blood supply to the various parts of visual pathway.

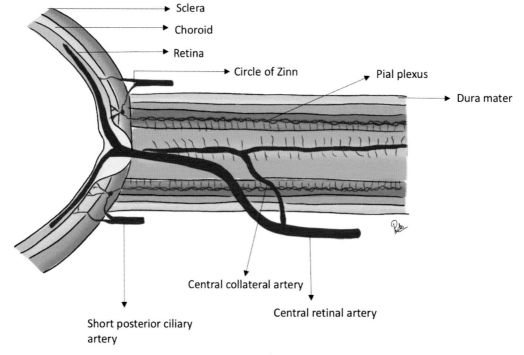

Fig. 1.20. The sheath and vascular supply to the intraocular and intraorbital portions of the optic nerve.

Pupillary Reflex

Shining light in one eye causes constriction of pupils in both eyes. Constriction of pupil in the eye where light in shone is called direct light reflex and constriction of pupil in the fellow eye is called consensual (indirect) light reflex

Pathway (Fig. 1.21)

- Afferent fibres travel along optic nerve and extend from retina to pretectal nucleus in mid brain at the level of superior colliculus
- At the optic chiasm, fibres from nasal retina decussate to optic tract on opposite side and terminate in contralateral pretectal nucleus. Fibres from the temporal retina remain uncrossed and terminate in ipsilateral pretectal nucleus
- Each pretectal nucleus is connected with Edinger Westphal nuclei of both sides via internuncial fibres (This forms the basis of consensual response)
- Parsympathetic fibres arising from Edinger-Westphal nucleus, travel along the oculomotor nerve (CN III) to form the efferent pathway
- Pre-ganglionic fibres travel along the inferior division of CN III and reach ciliary ganglion via nerve to inferior oblique
- Post-ganglionic fibres travel via short ciliary nerves to supply the sphincter pupillae causing constriction of pupil

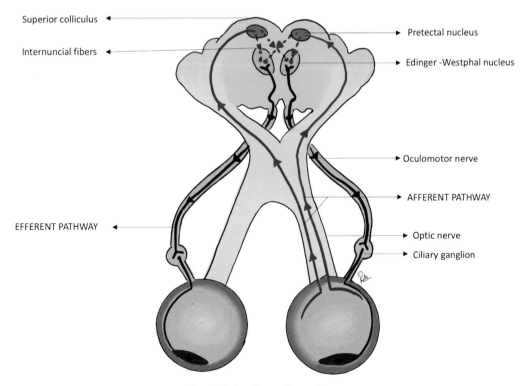

Fig. 1.21. Pupillary reflex pathway.

Take home messages

- The nerve fibres undergo decussation at the optic chiasm and it is an important landmark in localisation of lesions along the visual pathway.
- The visual fields are represented differently in the retina and at the visual cortex.

1.10 Selected Cranial Nerves Related to Ophthalmology

Learning Objectives
• Understand the pathway and function of the oculomotor, trochlear and abducen nerve.
• Learn the components and their relationship within the cavernous sinus.

Oculomotor Nerve (Cranial Nerve 3) (Fig. 1.22)

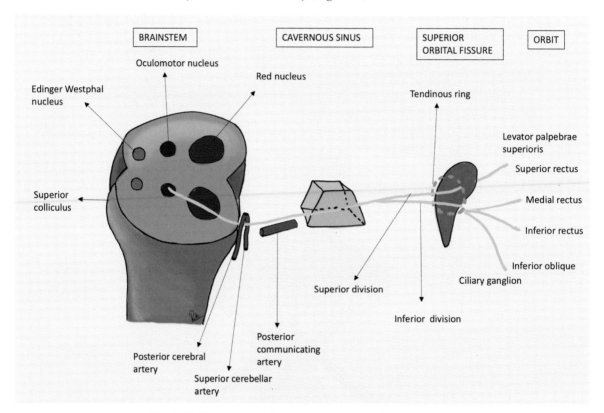

Fig. 1.22. Pictorial description of course of the oculomotor nerve.

• Oculomotor nuclei are found in the mid brain adjacent to the superior colliculi
• Passes anteriorly through the red nucleus and emerges on ventral side of mid brain where it lies between the posterior cerebral artery and the superior cerebellar artery
• Then it lies parallel to the posterior communicating artery (PCA), hence aneurysms of PCA may compress the nerve causing paresis
• Runs in the lateral wall of the cavernous sinus
• Divides into superior and inferior branches before entering the orbit via the superior orbital fissure
• All extraocular muscles except lateral rectus and superior oblique are supplied by the oculomotor nerve
• Inferior branch carries parasympathetic supply to ciliary ganglion

Trochlear Nerve (Cranial Nerve 4) (Fig. 1.23)

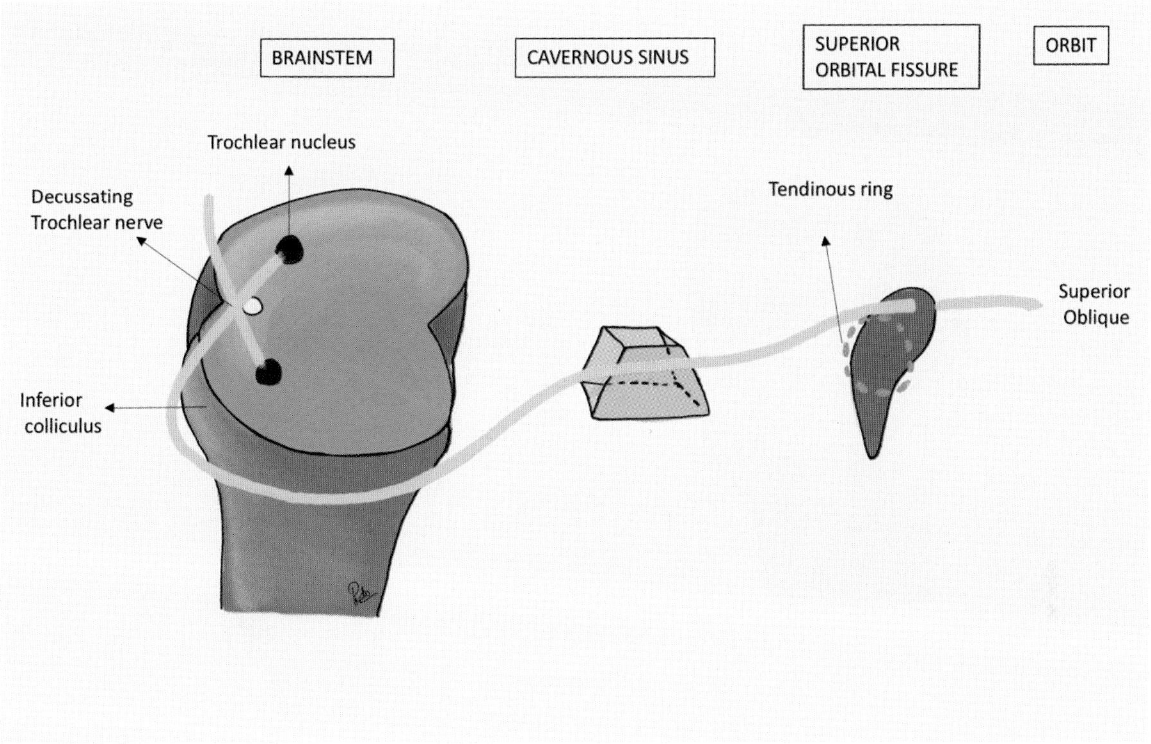

Fig. 1.23. Pictorial description of course of the trochlear nerve.

- Trochlear nerve nuclei are found in the mid-brain at the level of the inferior colliculus
- After emerging from nucleus, the fibres undergo decussation before exiting from the dorsal aspect of the brainstem. (hence supply the contralateral superior oblique muscle because of the decussation)
- It turns around the cerebral peduncles to enter the lateral wall of the cavernous sinus
- Enters the orbit through the superior orbital fissure lying outside the tendinous ring
- The trochlear nerve innervates the superior oblique muscle

Abducent Nerve (Cranial Nerve 6) (Fig. 1.24)

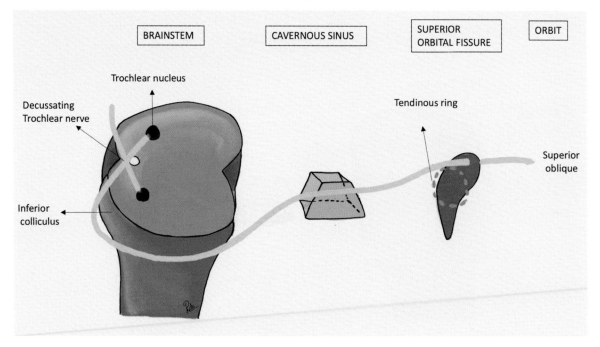

BRAINSTEM   CAVERNOUS SINUS   SUPERIOR ORBITAL FISSURE   ORBIT

Trochlear nucleus

Decussating Trochlear nerve

Tendinous ring

Superior oblique

Inferior colliculus

Fig. 1.24. Pictorial description of course of the abducent nerve.

- Nucleus lies at the level of the pons, ventral to the floor of the fourth ventricle. Facial nerve passes over it, forming the facial colliculus
- Emerges from the brainstem ventrally at the pontomedullary junction
- Passes up the clivus and over the apex of petrous part of temporal bone
- Then runs forward to lie wholly within the cavernous sinus. (Hence, it if often the first to be damages in cavernous sinus thrombosis.)
- Enters the orbit through the superior orbital fissure lying inside the common tendinous ring
- Supplies the lateral rectus muscle in the orbit

Facial Nerve (Cranial Nerve 7) (Fig. 1.25)

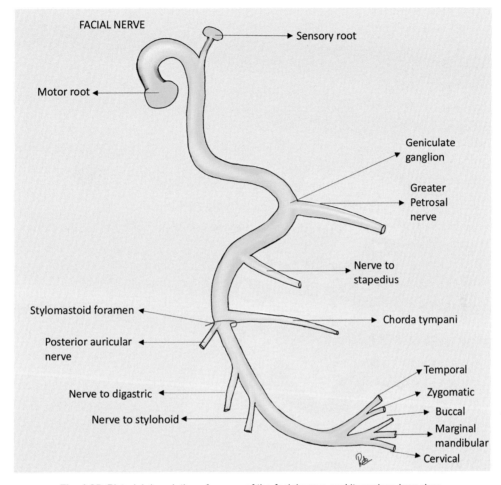

Fig. 1.25. Pictorial description of course of the facial nerve and its various branches.

- Nerve arises from pons as 2 roots: large motor root and small sensory root
- It emerges from brainstem ventrally between midbrain and pons after looping around the abducent nucleus
- 2 roots travel through the internal acoustic meatus
- After leaving the meatus, enters z-shaped facial canal
- Within the facial canal:
  - The 2 roots fuse
  - Nerve forms geniculate ganglion
  - The nerve gives rise to greater petrosal nerve, nerve to stapedius and chorda tympani
- Exits the facial canal through stylomastoid foramen
- Turns superiorly and runs anterior to outer ear. Gives rise to posterior auricular nerve, nerve to digastric and stylohyoid
- Within the parotid gland the nerve terminates by splitting into 5 terminal motor branches:
  - Temporal — supplies frontalis, orbicularis oculi and corrugator supercilii

- Zygomatic — supplies orbicularis oculi
- Buccal — supplies orbicularis oculi, buccinators and zygomaticus
- Marginal mandibular — supplies mentalis
- Cervical — supplies platysma

Cavernous Sinus

- Cavernous sinuses are located on either side of the body of sphenoid bone

Important contents and relations of cavernous sinus (Fig. 1.26):

- Extends from superior orbital fissure anteriorly to apex of petrous part of temporal bone posteriorly
- Floor is formed by dural covering of greater wing of sphenoid
- Medially related to pituitary fossa above the sphenoid sinus
- The internal carotid artery traverses upwards and forwards through the sinus, grooving the medial wall of the sinus
- Abducent nerve travels within the sinus. It is often the first structure damaged in cavernous sinus thrombosis
- The lateral wall encloses oculomotor nerve, trochlear nerve and first 2 divisions of trigeminal nerve
- Tributaries of cavernous sinus:
  - Superior ophthalmic vein
  - Inferior ophthalmic vein
  - Superficial middle cerebral veins
  - Inferior cerebral veins
  - Sphenoparietal sinus

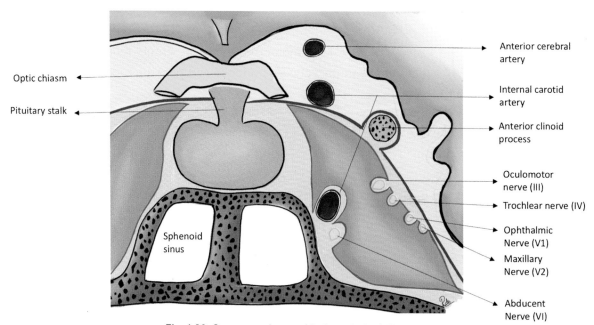

Fig. 1.26. Cavernous sinus and its important relations.

– Drainage of cavernous sinus is via superior and inferior petrosal sinus as well as venous plexus around internal carotid artery and emissary veins through skull base foramina

– Interconnections exist between the right and left cavernous sinuses. Hence, infection of one side can spread and manifest in the opposite side

Take home messages

• All extraocular muscles except lateral rectus and superior oblique are supplied by the oculomotor nerve.

• The trochlear nerve innervates the superior oblique muscle.

• The abducen nerve supplies the lateral rectus muscle.

• Infection in cavernous sinus can spread to opposite side.

References

1. American Academy of Ophthalmology — *Fundamentals and Principles of Ophthalmology.*

2. Snell R. *Clinical Anatomy of the Eye.*

Chapter 2

CORNEA AND EXTERNAL EYE DISEASES

2.1 Basic Anterior Segment Examination

Learning Objectives
- Recognising and understanding common corneal pathologies.
- Recognising normal and pathological slit-lamp examination findings.
- Ability to incorporate clinical findings with various common pathological cornea and external eye conditions.

Anterior segment examination can be performed grossly with the use of a torch light or direct ophthalmoscope. However, detailed examination would require the proficient use of the slit-lamp biomicroscopy (Fig. 2.1). A good understanding of the anterior segment anatomy is essential for identification of the various structures seen on the slit-lamp biomicroscopy. (Refer to Chapter on "Anterior Segment Anatomy"; Fig. 2.2.).

Slit-lamp Examination Findings based on Anatomy

	Findings to Look Out for
Conjunctival	Injection Nodules/growth (pinguecula, pterygium)
Cornea	Epithelial erosions/abrasions Scars Infiltrates Cornea oedema Cornea vascularisation
Anterior chamber	Anterior chamber depth Anterior chamber reaction — cells, flare Keratic precipitates
Iris	Nodules Atrophy Synechiae (peripheral anterior synechiae, posterior synechiae) Vascularisation Abnormal pupil (corectopia, polycoria)

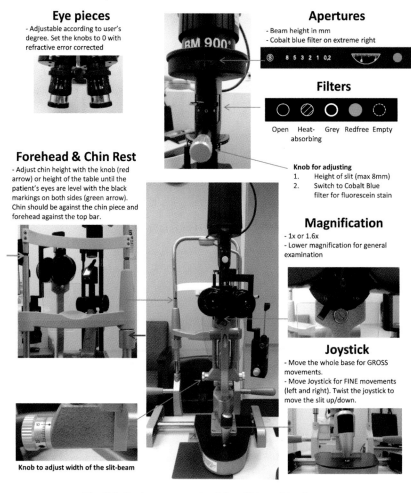

Eye pieces
- Adjustable according to user's degree. Set the knobs to 0 with refractive error corrected

Apertures
- Beam height in mm
- Cobalt blue filter on extreme right

Filters

Open   Heat-absorbing   Grey   Redfree   Empty

Forehead & Chin Rest
- Adjust chin height with the knob (red arrow) or height of the table until the patient's eyes are level with the black markings on both sides (green arrow). Chin should be against the chin piece and forehead against the top bar.

Knob for adjusting
1. Height of slit (max 8mm)
2. Switch to Cobalt Blue filter for fluorescein stain

Magnification
- 1x or 1.6x
- Lower magnification for general examination

Joystick
- Move the whole base for GROSS movements.
- Move Joystick for FINE movements (left and right). Twist the joystick to move the slit up/down.

Knob to adjust width of the slit-beam

Fig. 2.1. Basic components of the slit-lamp biomicroscope.

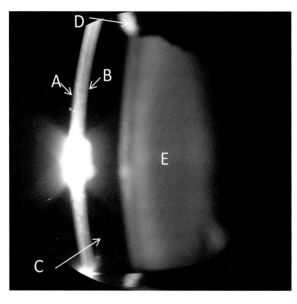

Fig. 2.2. Slit-beam image of the anterior segment demonstrating: (A) anterior corneal surface, (B) posterior corneal surface; (C) anterior chamber; (D) iris; and (E) cataract.

What are the Causes of a Red Eye?

	Ocular Causes	Extraocular Causes
Infective causes	Conjunctivitis Infective keratitis Endophthalmitis	Orbital cellulitis
Non-infective causes	Corneal abrasion Allergic conjunctivitis Blepharo-conjunctivitis Marginal keratitis Uveitis Acute primary angle closure Episcleritis Scleritis Dry eyes Subconjunctival haemorrhage	Thyroid eye disease Carotid-cavernous sinus Fistula

What are the Uses of Fluorescein Stain?

- Checking of intraocular pressure with Goldmann applanation tonometry
- Fluorescein dye disappearance test
- Stains epithelial defects and epitheliopathy
- To check for "tear break-up time"
- Reduction in tear break-up time seen in dry eyes
- To check for wound leak ("Seidel's" test)
- Hard contact lens fitting

What Causes a Diffusely Hazy Cornea?

- Raised intraocular pressure (e.g. acute primary angle closure)
- Bullous keratopathy from endothelial failure

Hazy cornea can be identified based on the inability to check the iris details and the pupil margin. Comparison with the fellow eye can be made in unilateral cases.

What are the Causes of a Focal Corneal Opacity?

- Infective keratitis
- Marginal keratitis
- Shield ulcer
- Corneal scar
    - Characterised by a quiescent eye — white conjunctiva, no surrounding corneal haze and no associated epithelial defect

Take home messages
- Not all red eyes are caused by viral conjunctivitis.
- Not all corneal opacities are infective in origin.

2.2 Subconjunctival Haemorrhage

Learning Objectives
• Recognise the appearance of subconjunctival haemorrhage.
• Management of subconjunctival haemorrhage.

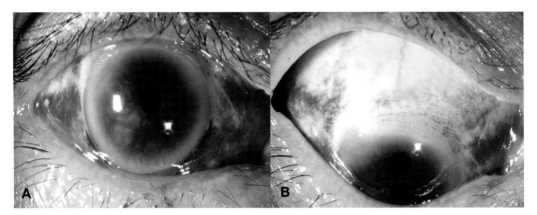

Fig. 2.3. Demonstrating subconjunctival haemorrhage of the eye at postoperative day 1 after a cataract surgery.

What is a Subconjunctival Haemorrhage?
• Occurs due to a rupture of the conjunctival vessels
• Results in a homogenous red patch on the conjunctiva (Fig. 2.3)

What are the Risk Factors for this Occurring?
• Trauma
• Blood thinners (e.g. aspirin, warfarin, clopidogrel)
• Hypertension
• Valsalva manoeuvre (e.g. constipation, coughing)

What is the Typical History?
• Sudden onset of red eye
• Painless
• No associated blurring of vision
• May have associated risk factors

What History or Clinical Finding are you Concerned About?
• Trauma
  ▪ Will need to exclude underlying scleral involvement
• Unable to see posterior extent of subconjunctival haemorrhage
  ▪ Need to rule out retrobulbar haemorrhage

How would you Manage the Patient?

- Conservative
  - Reassurance. Majority are managed conservatively and will resolve in 1–2 weeks spontaneously
- Further management is dependent on the presence of other ocular injuries

In a patient with no risk factors and recurrent subconjunctival haemorrhage, consider working up for haematological abnormalities.

Take home messages
Subconjunctival haemorrhage is very common and it is important to rule out severe trauma.

2.3 Corneal Infections

Learning Objectives
- Recognise the signs and symptoms of infective keratitis.
- Understanding the acute management of infective keratitits.

Infective keratitis can result from various types of organisms including viral, bacterial, fungal, parasitic. Viral, fungal and parasitic infections tend to occur more commonly in the immunosuppressed individuals, while bacterial infections occur in those with other preexisting risk factors. Contact lens use, ocular contact with contaminated water or solution, corneal trauma and prolonged topical steroid use are the main risk factors for many of these infections.

Table 2.1. Examples of Various Aetiological Causes of Infective Keratitis

Viral	Herpes simplex virus 1 Herpes simplex virus 2 Varicella zoster virus
Bacterial	*Pseudomonas aeruginosa* *Staphylococcus aureus* Streptococcus species Atypical bacteria (e.g. Mycobacterium species)
Fungal	Candida species Fusarium species
Parasitic	Microsporidia Acanthamoeba species

Herpetic Keratitis

What is Herpetic Keratitis?
- Herpetic infection of the cornea
- Can affect various layers of the cornea
- Primarily caused by herpes simplex virus 1 (more commonly) and 2

- Virus can remain dormant in the trigeminal nerve and manifest with frequent reactivation
- Ocular manifestations are the result of ocular inflammation, viral activity, or both

What are the Symptoms that Patient may Present with?

- Red eye
- Pain or ocular irritation
- Tearing
- Photophobia

What are the Clinical Signs?

- Reduced corneal sensation
- Conjunctival injection
- Epithelial keratitis may present with dendritic or geographic ulcers which will stain with fluorescein (Fig. 2.4 and Fig. 2.5)
  - Dendritic ulcers are seen typically as branching lesions with terminal bulbs
  - Multiple dendritic ulcers coalesce to form a geographic ulcer
- Stromal infiltration and corneal oedema may be present in stromal keratitis
- Anterior chamber reaction may be present in herpetic keratouveitis or endothelitis

Healing corneal abrasions can present as "pseudo-dendrites" and are frequently misdiagnosed as herpetic epithelial keratitis.

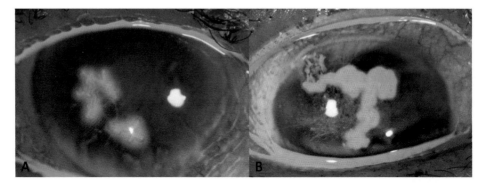

Fig. 2.4. Photographs demonstrating epithelial keratitis with dendritic ulcer seen in (A) and a geographic ulcer seen in (B).

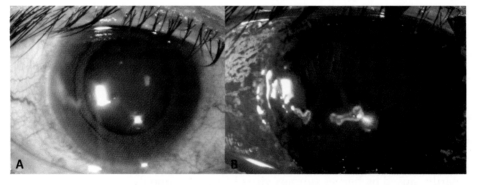

Fig. 2.5. Photographs demonstrating dendritic ulcer before (A) and after (B) fluorescein staining.

What are the Risk Factors for this Condition?

- Reduced host immunity (e.g. HIV, organ transplant recipient, pregnancy)
- Long-term immunosuppression (e.g. systemic or topical steroids)
- Recent ocular surgery

How do we Manage these Patients?

- Depends on the level of the corneal involvement
- Patients are generally started on antiviral treatment such as topical acyclovir
- In the presence of stromal/endothelial keratitis, topical steroids must be added
- Oral acyclovir may be started in immunocompromised patients or children with HSV keratitis
- Oral acyclovir 400 mg twice a day can be started for long-term prophylactic treatment of recurrent herpetic keratitis

Topical steroids should be avoided in the presence of epithelial keratitis.

What are the Possible Long-term Complications?

- Recurrence
- Neurotrophic keratopathy with persistent epithelial defect or ulcer
- Stromal scarring
  - Resulting in high irregular astigmatism
  - Dense scarring may require treatment with corneal transplant

What are the Other Ocular Manifestations of Herpes Simplex Virus?

- Blepharitis
- Acute anterior uveitis
- Retinitis
- Cranial nerve palsies

HSV blepharitis can present as a focal area of vesicular rash over the eyelid. This does not follow a dermatomal pattern as seen in HZO.

Herpes Zoster Ophthalmicus

What is Herpes Zoster Oophthalmicus?

- Caused by reactivation of varicella zoster virus
- Manifests as a painful vesicular rash along the ophthalmic division (V1) of the trigeminal nerve distribution
- Vesicles or pustules eventually crust and heal within 2–6 weeks

What are the Important Examination Findings?

- Vesicular or pustular rash seen along the V1 dermatome distribution (some may be crusting)
- Look for involvement of the tip of the nose
- Check corneal sensation

- Visual acuity
- Intraocular pressure
  - Raised intraocular pressure may occur secondary to ocular inflammation
- Slit-lamp examination
  - Conjunctival injection
  - Stain the cornea to look for dendritic lesions
    - i. Typically without terminal bulbs and without central ulceration
  - Anterior chamber reaction seen in keratouveitis
- Dilated fundus examination looking for posterior segment involvement

What is Hutchinson's Sign? (Fig. 2.6)

- This is when there is involvement of the tip of the nose
- Indicates involvement of the nasociliary branch of V1 of the trigeminal nerve
- This increases the risk of corneal involvement (50–76% chance of ocular complications)

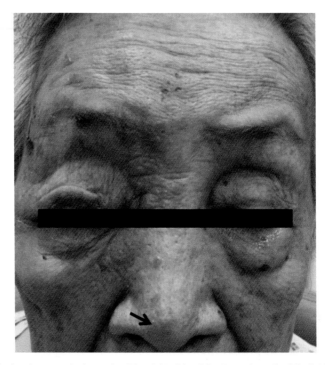

Fig. 2.6. Photograph showing a vesicular rash of the right side of the face along the V1 distribution. Hutchinson's sign is positive (shown by arrow).

What are Some of the Risk Factors?

- Advanced age
- Psychological stress
- Immuno suppressed state (e.g. systemic steroids)
- Immuno compromised patient (e.g. HIV, malignancies)

How would you Manage the Patient?

- Isolate the patient
- Start oral acyclovir 800 mg 5 times a day for 2 weeks
- Start acyclovir ointment to the eye 5 times a day if there is corneal involvement
- Topical antibiotic cream to skin lesions to reduce risk of secondary bacterial infection
- May require steroid eyedrops if there is associated ocular inflammation

When there are multiple dermatomal involvement or multiple recurrences, always consider an immunocompromised state. Further blood investigations may be warranted.

What are the Possible Long-term Complications?

- Neurotrophic keratopathy due to impaired corneal innervation
- Post-herpetic neuralgia (10–17%)

Bacterial Keratitis

What are the common Organisms for Bacterial Keratitis?

- *Pseudomonas aeruginosa*
- Staphylococcus
- Streptococcus

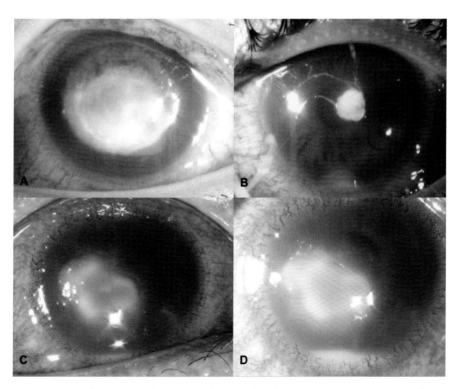

Fig. 2.7. (A, B) Demonstrating central corneal ulcer secondary to *Pseudomonas aeruginosa* with a clump of hypopyon seen in (B). (C) Demonstates a central corneal ulcer with a hypopyon secondary to polymicrobial keratitis without fluorescein staining, and (D) with fluorescein staining, demonstrating an overlying epithelial defect.

What are the Risk Factors?

- Contact lens — poor contact lens hygiene, overnight contact lens wear, contaminated contact lens solution
- Trauma
- Contaminated water contact with the eye

What are the Other Organisms that can Cause a Corneal Ulcer?

- Viral (e.g. herpetic)
- Fungal (e.g. fusarium, candida)
- Atypical organisms — mycobacterium, acanthoameba

What are the Clinical Signs? (Fig. 2.7)

- Conjunctival injection
- Corneal infiltrate
- Epithelial defect
- Hypopyon
- Anterior chamber reaction

How would you Manage the Patient?

- Corneal scraping to send for gram stain, fungal smear, fungal culture, aerobic and anaerobic culture
- May consider sending the contact lens/solution for culture
- Start hourly fortified topical cefazolin 50 mg/mL and topical gentamicin 14 mg/mL
- Topical cycloplegia

What are the Possible Complications?

- Corneal melt and perforation
- Corneal scar

Take home messages

- Contact lens wear, contaminated water or solution, ocular trauma and prolonged use of topical steroids are the main risk factors for infective keratitis.
- Early diagnosis and targeted treatment is important to reduce sight-threatening complications and scarring.
- Topical steroids should be avoided in the initial treatment of infective keratitis.

2.4 Conjunctivitis

Learning Objectives

- Recognising and understanding the various causes for conjunctivitis.
- Management of the various causes of conjunctivitis.

Conjunctivitis is an inflammation of the conjunctiva which can be due to various causes. It is important to recognise the diagnosis as this has direct implications on the management of the patient. For example, failing to recognise an episode of allergic conjunctivitis can result in delayed treatment and recurrent flares.

Allergic Conjunctivitis

What are the Types of Allergic Conjunctivitis?

- Seasonal/perennial conjunctivitis
- Atopic keratoconjunctivitis (AKC)
- Vernal keratoconjunctivitis (VKC)

What are the Differences between the Various Types of Allergic Conjunctivitis?

	Seasonal	VKC	AKC
Epidemiology		Typically aged 5–20 years old Predominantly in male	Teenage to 50-years old Chronic course with periodic acute exacerbations.
Hypersensitivity reaction	Type 1	Type 1 and 4	Type 4
Associations	May have other atopy	May not have history of atopy Keratoconus (from rubbing)	High association with atopic dermatitis and asthma Increased risk with positive family history Keratoconus Anterior/posterior subcapsular cataracts
Symptoms	Seasonal symptoms from environmental allergens (pollens, animal dander) Rapid symptoms after exposure (short lived and episodic)	Seasonal variation Environmental allergen may incite acute exacerbation	Disease year round Relapses and remits without seasonal correlation
Examination findings	Generally no corneal involvement	Limbal and palpabral form Giant papillae of **only superior tarsal conjunctival** Limbal (Horner Trantas dots) Corneal vernal plaques or shield (Togby's) ulcer	Papillary hypertrophy of **superior and inferior** tarsal conjunctival with increased risk of eyelid thickening and scarring

What is the Typical History?

- Intense itch
- Intermittent red eyes
- Lid swelling
- Thick ropy mucoid discharge

What are the Clinical Signs? (Fig. 2.8)

- Conjunctival chemosis
- Conjunctival injection
- Epithelial erosions or epithelial defect
- Papillae or cobblestone papillae
- Horner trantas dots or limbitis
- Shield ulcer

What are the Chronic Eye Changes that can Occur with Untreated VKC or AKC? (Fig. 2.9)

- Loss of eyelashes
- Conjunctival scarring
- Corneal neovascularisation
- Corneal ulcer
- Corneal scarring
- Keratoconus

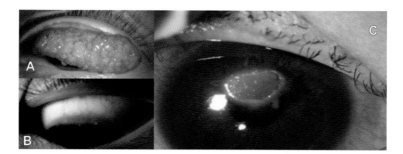

Fig. 2.8. Demonstrating various clinical signs seen in vernal keratoconjunctivitis such as (A) cobblestone papillae, (B) limbitis, and (C) shield ulcer.

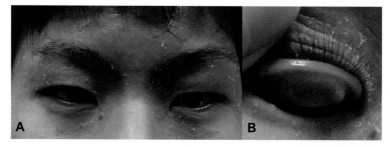

Fig. 2.9. Demonstrating a case of atopic keratoconjunctivitis with (A) periocular dermatitis, and (B) papillae seen upon lid eversion.

What are Shield Ulcers?

- Sterile ulcers or plaques are macro-erosions that form due to accumulation of fibrin and mucous
- Typically located at the upper 2/3 of the cornea

> Shield ulcers are not infective in nature. Unlike infective keratitis, treatment will require the use of topical steroids while preventing secondary infection with topical antibiotics.

What are the Risk Factors?

- Atopic history of asthma, allergic rhinitis or eczema
- Young, male

What may Exacerbate Symptoms?

- House dustmites
- Dander
- Contact lens
- Dry eyes

How would you Manage this Patient?

- Systemic management
  - Allergen avoidance
  - Skin prick test
  - Control of other allergies
- Ocular management
  - Topical mast cell stabilisers
  - Topical anti-histamines
  - Topical lubricants
  - Cold compress
  - Topical steroids
  - Topical immunomodulators — cyclosporin, tacrolimus
  - Systemic steroids in severe cases
  - Supratarsal injection of steroid for recalcitrant cases

Viral Conjunctivitis

What is the most Common Causative Virus?

- Adenovirus

What History does the Patient Present with? (Fig. 2.10)

- Sequential red eyes
- Sticky discharge
- Tearing
- Other history — recent upper respiratory tract infection, lymphadenopathy, contact history

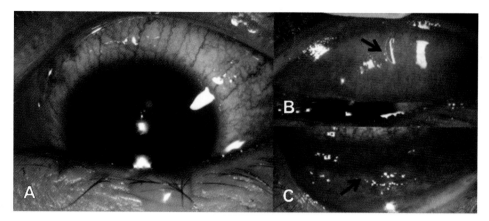

Fig. 2.10. Demonstrating various clinical signs seen in viral conjunctivitis, such as (A) diffuse conjunctival injection, (B) pseudomembrane seen on upper lid eversion, and (C) follicular conjunctival reaction on lower lid eversion.

What are the Clinical Findings?

- Conjunctival injection
- Conjunctival follicular reaction
- Pseudomembranes seen on lid eversion
- Check for corneal involvement — punctate epitheliopathy, epithelial defect

What are the Other Causes of Conjunctivitis?

- Bacterial conjunctivitis
  - Consider if extensive purulent discharge
  - Multiple sexual partners
- Allergic conjunctivitis
  - Chronic intermittent history of red eyes
  - Associated with itch predominantly
  - Background of other atopies
- Toxic conjunctivitis
  - Chronic use of topical eyedrops

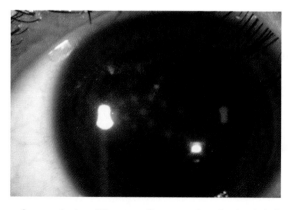

Fig. 2.11. A case of nummular keratitits seen after an acute episode of viral conjunctivitis.

How would you Manage the Patient?

- Topical lubricants
- Generally self-limiting over 1–2 weeks
- Advise patient to practise good hand hygiene as viral conjunctivitis is highly contagious

What are the Possible Complications?

- Corneal epitheliopathy or epithelial defect
- Nummular keratitis (Fig. 2.11)

Take home messages
- Not every red eye is viral conjunctivitis!
- Take a detailed history, in particular, the presence of known atopy.
- There are various types of allergic conjunctivitis depending on their presentation. However, the principle of management is similar.

2.5 Corneal Transplant

Learning Objectives
- Basic understanding of indications for a corneal transplant.
- Recognising the presence of a corneal transplant graft.

Corneal transplants have evolved over the years from primarily performing full thickness graft, to replacing only the diseased part of the cornea through performing a partial thickness keratoplasty. However, this involves overcoming a greater learning curve.

Comparable visual outcomes can be achieved after a lamellar keratoplasty, with improvement in graft survival, reduced rejection rates and postoperative glaucoma reported after a penetrating keratoplasty. Posterior lamellar keratoplasty allows for faster visual recovery with reduced risk of sight-threatening intraoperative complications such as suprachoroidal haemorrhage.

What are the Types of Corneal Transplants? (Fig. 2.12)

- Full thickness
  - Penetrating keratoplasty
- Partial thickness
  - Anterior lamellar keratoplasty
  - Endothelial keratoplasty
- Corneal patch graft

What are the Common Indications for a Corneal Transplant?

- Optical indications
  - Corneal scar
  - Keratoconus

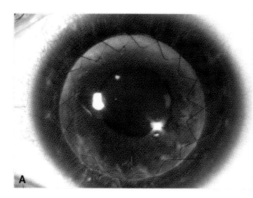 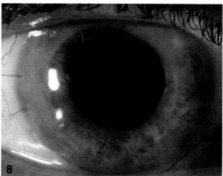

Fig. 2.12. Of an eye post-corneal transplant: (A) After deep anterior lamellar keratoplasty, and (B) After endothelial keratoplasty.

- Bullous keratopathy
- Corneal dystrophy
- Tectonic indication
  - Corneal perforation
- Therapeutic indication
  - Severe infective keratitis refractory to medical treatment

What are the Possible Complications of a Corneal Transplant?

- Glaucoma
- Infection
- Graft rejection
- Graft failure

Take home messages

- Different types of corneal transplant is performed depending on the location of the pathology.
- Penetrating keratoplasty → full thickness corneal scar.
- Endothelial keratoplasty → bullous keratopathy.
- Anterior lamellar keratoplasty → keratoconus, corneal scars.

2.6 Pterygium

Learning Objectives

- Recognising a pterygium and understanding the clinical consequences of the condition.
- Understanding common differentials such as a pseudopterygium and a pinguecula (Fig. 2.13).

Pterygium is a fibrovascular, wing-shaped growth of the conjunctiva over the cornea. It is typically located at the interpalpabral region (3- and 9 o'clock) position and is degenerative in nature (Fig. 2.14).

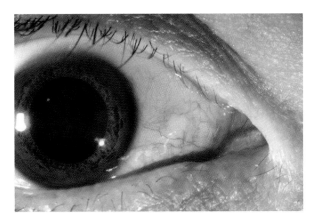

Fig. 2.13. Nasal pinguecula seen as a raised yellow-white conjunctival lesion. This is similarly secondary to UV exposure.

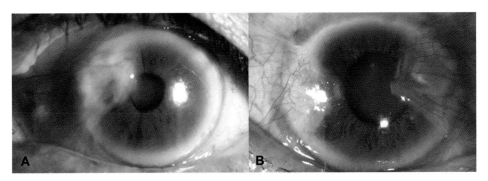

Fig. 2.14. Demonstrating (A) Nasal pterygium, and a (B) Double-headed pterygium.

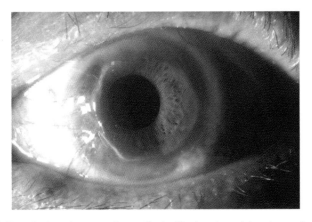

Fig. 2.15. Pseudopterygium seen in a patient with chronic peripheral ucerative keratitis.

Suspect a pseudopterygium in the presence of a unilateral lesion NOT located at the interpalpabral region. This may be due to a previous insult (e.g. chemical injury) or chronic ocular inflammation (Fig. 2.15).

What are the Risk Factors?

- Sunlight exposure (main risk factor)
- Dry eyes
- Dust exposure

What are the Clinical Consequences?

- Majority asymptomatic
- Dry eyes related symptoms from irregular ocular surface
- Induced corneal astigmatism
- Obstruction of visual axis
- Cosmesis

What are Indications for Surgery?

- Visual axis is involved
- High astigmatism
- Cosmesis

How would you Manage the Patient?

- Most pterygiums can be treated conservatively. Sunglasses can be worn to reduce sunlight exposure
- Surgery is performed if clinically significant. Patient can undergo pterygium excision with conjunctival autograft

In a patient with a significant pterygium and a concomitant cataract, the pterygium is usually removed first to reduce the induced astigmatism before planning for cataract surgery.

Take home messages

Pterygium is a common degenerative condition and may be managed conservatively if it is not causing any symptoms.

2.7 Episcleritis and Scleritis

Learning Objectives

- Recognising the difference between episcleritis and scleritis.
- Understanding the necessary investigations and management in these cases.

Episcleritis is an inflammation of the superficial episcleral vessels of the eye. On the other hand, scleritis involves inflammation of the deeper scleral vessels. It is important to differentiate between the two conditions as episcleritis is generally benign, while scleritis requires further systemic investigations. It is necessary to rule out autoimmune conditions in these cases, which may require subsequent systemic treatment.

What are the Types of Episcleritis and Scleritis?

Episcleritis	Scleritis

• Diffuse
• Sectoral
• Nodular
	• Anterior
	 • Non-necrotising
	   i. Diffuse
	   ii. Nodular
	 • Necrotising
	   i. Inflammatory
	   ii. Non-inflammatory (Scleromalacia perforans)
	• Posterior

What History would the Patient Present with?

- Red eye
- Scleritis can present as an eye pain that is worse with eye movements and may wake the patient up at night
- May have a history of previous episodes
- History of autoimmune conditions
- Typically no discharge or infective symptoms

What are the Clinical Findings?

- Episcleritis
  - Diffuse, sectoral or nodular injection
  - Episcleral vessels seen mobile over underlying scleral
  - May have anterior chamber reaction
- Scleritis
  - Bluish-red violaceous hue (best seen under daylight) (Fig. 2.16)
  - Scleral tenderness
  - May have anterior chamber reaction
  - Look for signs of previous ocular surgery (e.g. previous pterygium excision or corneal wound)
    - i. Surgically induced necrotising scleritis
  - Dilate the fundus to check for posterior segment inflammation (e.g. choroidal folds, disc swelling, serous retinal detachment)

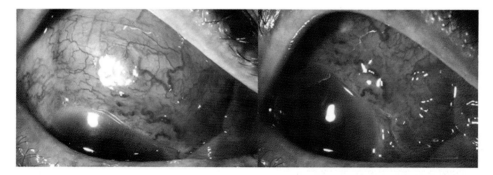

Fig. 2.16. Demonstrating a case of nodular scleritis.

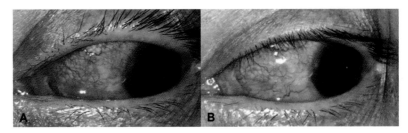

Fig. 2.17. Demonstrating a case of scleritis (A) before, and (B) after, phenylephrine 2.5% instillation. There is absence of blanching of the deep scleral vessels.

What is the Clinical Test to Differenciate between Episcleritis and Scleritis?

- Phenylephrine 2.5% is used to blanch the overlying conjunctival and episcleral vessels (Fig. 2.17)
- Absence of blanching of the deep scleral vessels is seen in scleritis

What Investigations would you Perform?

- Episcleritis
  - Mostly idiopathic
  - Systemic evaluation only necessary in recurrent episodes
- Scleritis
  - B scan ultrasonography to look for "T sign" due to fluid in subtenon space
  - Systemic workup to rule out infective and autoimmune conditions
    - i. Full blood count, erythrocyte sedimentation rate, rheumatoid factor, anti-nuclear antibody, lupus screen, anti-neutrophil cytoplasmic antibody and urine microscopy looking for hematuria
    - ii. Chest X-ray, Mantoux test, syphilis screen

How would you Manage the Patient?

- Episcleritis — topical NSAIDs or topical steroids
- Anterior scleritis
  - Topical NSAID and oral NSAIDS
  - May consider oral steroids
  - Necrotising scleritis may require pulse Intravenous steroid treatment
- Posterior scleritis — Systemic steroids

What are the Possible Complications of Scleritis?

- Necrotising anterior scleritis can present with scleral thinning and perforation
- Raised intraocular pressure
- Serous retinal detachment

Take home messages

- It is important to differenciate episcleritis and scleritis since scleritis requires further investigations and systemic treatment.
- Scleritis can lead to sight-threatening complications and requires early diagnosis and treatment.

2.8 Anterior Segment Trauma

Learning Objectives
• Recognising and understanding various types of anterior segment trauma.
• Understanding the acute management of types of ocular trauma.

Ocular trauma can be either sharp or blunt in nature. Depending on the mechanism, the location and severity of the injury, there are various acute and long-term implications to the management of the patient. The Birmingham Eye Trauma Terminology system (BETT) provides a classification of the various types of ocular injuries and the ocular trauma score allows us to prognosticate the injury (Fig. 2.18).

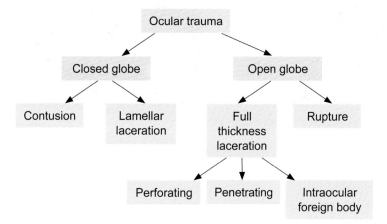

Fig. 2.18. Birmingham Eye Trauma Terminology system.

Table 2.2. Prognostication Factors in the Ocular Trauma Score

• Presenting visual acuity
• Presence of
  i. Globe rupture
  ii. Endophthalmitis
  iii. Perforating Injury
  iv. Retinal detachment
  v. Relative afferent pupillary defect

Corneal Abrasion

What is the Typical History?
• Preceding trauma
• Pain and tearing
• Inability to open the eye
• Red eye

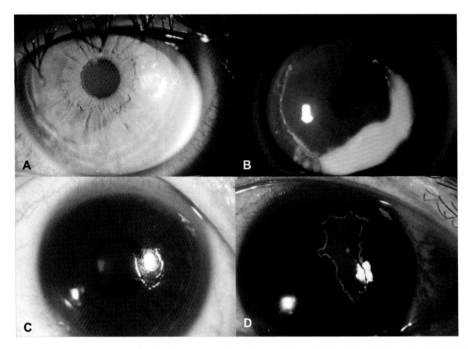

Fig. 2.19. Demonstrating a corneal abrasion seen without fluorescein staining (A and C), and with fluorescein staining under cobalt blue light (B and D), respectively.

What are the Clinical Signs?

- Corneal epithelial defect that fluoresce under cobalt blue light when fluorescein stain is applied to the eye (Fig. 2.19)
- Important to rule out secondary infection
  - Look for corneal infiltrates and cellular activity

How would you Manage the Patient?

- Lubricants
  - Preservative free artificial teardrops
  - Ointment (e.g. Duratears)
- Topical antibiotics to prevent secondary infection

> A drop of topical tetracaine prior to examination will make the patient more comfortable. DO NOT discharge the patient with tetracaine drops as that can cause epithelial toxicity instead.

What are the Potential Long-term Complications?

- Corneal scar
- Recurrent corneal abrasion

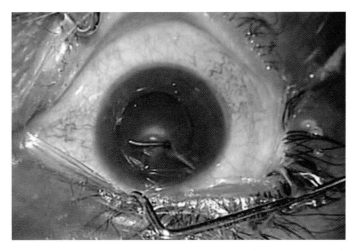

Fig. 2.20. Demonstrating an ocular penetrating injury secondary to a foreign body. The foreign body is seen lodged within the cornea.

Corneal Laceration

What are the Common Mechanisms of Injury?
- Rupture
  - Blunt trauma (e.g. golf ball injury)
  - High pressure injury (e.g. hydraulic-injection injury)
- Laceration (Fig. 2.20)
  - High velocity injury (e.g. grinding metal) — suspect intraocular foreign body if entry wound seen
  - Sharp injury (e.g. scissors, wires, hammering of nail)

What is your Immediate Management?
- Ensure the patient is hemodynamically stable — Ensure "Airway, Breathing, Circulation" intact
- Keep the patient "Nil by mouth"
- IM tetanus
- IV ciprofloxacin
- Keep an eye shield on
  - Do not touch the eye further as that may lead to further damage of intraocular structures and worsen the prognosis
- Refer to ophthalmology for subsequent assessment and surgical repair of corneal laceration and associated injuries

Do not pull out a foreign body lodged within the laceration in an open globe injury. This should be done in a controlled manner in the operating theatre.

What Investigations will you Perform?

- Arrange for a CT orbits (1 mm fine cuts) to rule out intraocular foreign body

What are the Poor Prognostic Factors in an Ocular Trauma?

- Poor presenting visual acuity
- Presence of relative afferent papillary defect
- Retinal detachment
- Globe rupture
- Endophthalmitis
- Perforating injury

Chemical Injury

What are the Types of Chemical Injuries and How do they Differ in Severity?

- Alkaline injury
  - More damaging as it saponifies lipids of cell membranes, penetrating deeper and more rapidly
- Acidic injury
  - Generally less damaging

What are the Important Clinical Findings that would Determine Severity and the Prognosis of the Injury?

- Extent of corneal abrasion
- Corneal haziness and clarity of iris details
- Extent of conjunctival involvement
- Limbal ischaemia (Fig. 2.21)

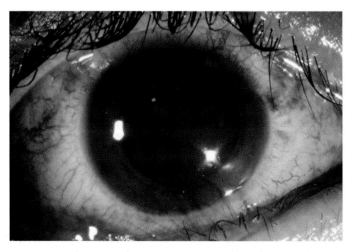

Fig. 2.21. Demonstrating a total corneal abrasion after an alkaline splash injury. Limbal ischaemia is seen from 3–8 o'clock position.

How would you Manage the Patient Acutely?

- Remove the inciting factor
  - Irrigate the eye immediately with at least 1 litre of normal saline. Check the pH (ensure pH7) and irrigate further if necessary
  - Evert the lids to remove gross debris
- Promote re-epithelialisation
  - Generous amount of lubricants with hourly preservative free eyedrops, and ointments
  - May require use of bandage contact lens or amniotic membrane transplant in the presence of persistent epithelial defect
- Reduce ocular inflammation with a short course of topical steroid (not more than 10 days)
- Topical antibiotics to prevent secondary infection
- Treat any associated complications such as acute rise in intra-ocular pressure

What are the Long-term Complications?

- Persistent inflammation
- Persistent epithelial defect or recurrent epithelial breakdown
- Glaucoma
- Lid abnormalities (e.g. trichiasis, dystichiasis, entropion)
- Cataract

Hyphema

What is a Hyphema?

- Fluid level of blood seen in the anterior chamber (Fig. 2.22)
- Due to rupture of iris or angle vessels

What Important History you would take from the Patient?

- Trauma (e.g. shuttlecock injury, punched)
- Ischaemic risk factors (e.g. DM, HTN)

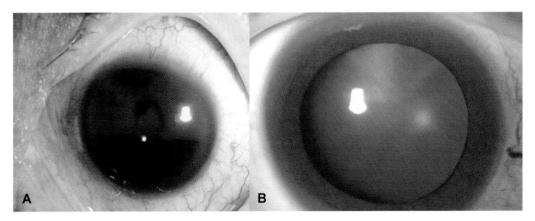

Fig. 2.22. (A) Hyphema as demonstrated by a dark red fluid level. (B) Shows iris neovascularisation in a patient secondary to proliferative diabetic retinopathy.

- Ocular history (e.g. recent surgery, chronic retinal detachment)
- History of haematological malignancies

What are the Risk Factors?

- Trauma
- Risk of iris neovascularisation (3 most important)
  - Proliferative diabetic retinopathy
  - Central retinal vein occlusion
  - Ocular ischemic syndrome

What are the Important Clinical Findings?

- Visual acuity
- Intraocular pressure
- Level of the hyphema (for monitoring)
- Look for iris neovascularisation and perform gonioscopy
- Dilated fundus examination looking for retinopathy
- In the presence of trauma, rule out other trauma-related injury

How would you Manage the Patient?

- Management dependent on underlying aetiology
- Trauma-related
  - Complete rest in bed
  - Sleep 45° to allow blood to settle inferiorly
  - Topical steroid
  - Topical cycloplegia
  - Topical anti-glaucoma medications if raised intraocular pressure
  - Monitor the patient closely for re-bleeding, raised intraocular pressure or corneal blood staining
- Non-trauma related
  - Manage underlying medical condition

What are the Complications of a Trauma-related Hyphema?

- Raised intraocular pressure
- Corneal blood staining
- Long term risk of angle recession glaucoma

Take home messages

- Ocular trauma requires early and prompt treatment to maximise visual prognosis.
- Long-term monitoring or prolonged visual rehabilitation may be required for many of these patients.

References

1. Borderie VM, Sandali O, Bullet J, *et al.* (2012) Long-term results of deep anterior lamellar versus penetrating keratoplasty. *Ophthalmology* **119**(2):249–55.

2. Han DC, Mehta JS, Por YM, *et al.* (2009) Comparison of outcomes of lamellar keratoplasty and penetrating keratoplasty in keratoconus. *AJ Ophthalmology* **148**(5):744–51.e1.

3. Lee WB, Jacobs DS, Musch DC, *et al.* (2009) Descemet's stripping endothelial keratoplasty: safety and outcomes: a report by the American Academy of Ophthalmology. *Ophthalmology* **116**(9):1818–30.

4. Kuhn F, Morris R, Witherspoon CD, *et al.* (1996) A standardized classification of ocular trauma. Graefe's archive for clinical and experimental ophthalmology. Albrecht von Graefes Archiv fur klinische und experimentelle Ophthalmologie **234**(6):399–403.

5. Kuhn F, Morris R, Witherspoon CD, *et al.* (2004) The Birmingham Eye Trauma Terminology system (BETT). Journal francais d'ophtalmologie **27**(2):206–10.

6. Scott R. (2015) The Ocular Trauma Score. *Community Eye Health* **28**(91):44–5.

Chapter 3

CATARACT

Learning Objectives
- Recognising the different types of cataracts and the clinical implications.
- Understanding the indications and principles of management of cataract.

Cataract is the opacification of our native lens. It can be due to various aetiologies of which degenerative causes are the most common. The lens opacity classification (LOCS III) (Fig. 3.1) can be used to categorise age-related cataracts according to their type and density. Management of visually significant cataracts is primarily through surgical removal.

3.1 Senile Cataract

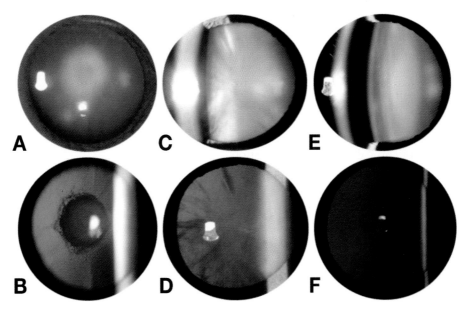

Fig. 3.1. Demonstrating posterior subcapsular cataract (A,B), cortical cataract (C,D), and nuclear sclerotic cataract (E,F).

What are the Causes of Cataract?

- Age-related
- Drug-related (e.g. steroid)
- Radiation-related
- Traumatic
- Congenital
- Metabolic

What are the Common Types of Cataracts?

- Cortical cataract
  - Can progress rapidly and cause more glare
- Posterior subcapsular cataract
  - Can progress rapidly and result in significant glare
- Nuclear sclerotic cataract
  - Associated with myopic shift

What is the Typical Presenting History?

- Progressive, painless, blurring of vision
- Change in refractive power
- Increase glare (especially posterior capsular and cortical cataracts)
- Altered contrast sensitivity

What are the Important Examination Findings?

- Relative afferent pupillary defect (RAPD)
  - Generally there should not be a RAPD if the cause of the blurring of vision is due to cataract
- Visual acuity
- Intraocular pressure
- Slit-lamp examination — density and type of cataract, anterior chamber depth, corneal dystrophy, corneal scar, lens subluxation
- Fundus examination (For visual prognosis)

When will you Offer Cataract Surgery?

- Visually significant cataract
  - Generally taken to be 6/12 or worse
  - Significant glare
- Secondary complications of cataract
  - Narrow angles, lens mechanism related glaucoma, subluxed lens

Consider the following before offering a patient surgery:
- Indication for the cataract surgery
- The functional impact of the cataract
  - Occupation
  - Hobbies
- The visual prognosis
- What are the visual requirements of the patient? Will the patient benefit from a mono-focal or multifocal lens?
- Is this a regular or complex case? What is the best surgical approach?
- Is the patient fit for surgery?

3.2 Principles of Management

What are the different types of cataract surgeries?
- Phacoemulsification (Fig. 3.2)
  - The emulsified lens is removed through a small 2–3mm wound. A foldable intraocular lens (IOL) is inserted through the small wound
  - Femtosecond laser may be used to assist in parts of the surgery (wound creation, capsulorhexis or lens fragmentation)
- Extracapsular cataract extraction (ECCE)
  - A large incision wound (about 10mm) is created and the entire cataract is delivered as a whole, while leaving the capsular bag intact
  - The IOL is placed within the capsular bag
  - Sutures are needed to close the large corneal wound
- Intracapsular cataract extraction (ICCE)
  - A large wound is created and the entire cataract is delivered together with the capsular bag
  - The IOL has to be placed in either the anterior chamber or be scleral-fixated

What is Phacoemulsification?
- Phacoemulsification involves the use of an ultrasonic probe that delivers energy into the eye to break up and emulsify a cataract

What are the Main Types of Intraocular Lenses?
- Monofocal IOL
- Multifocal IOL
- Toric IOL for astigmatic correction

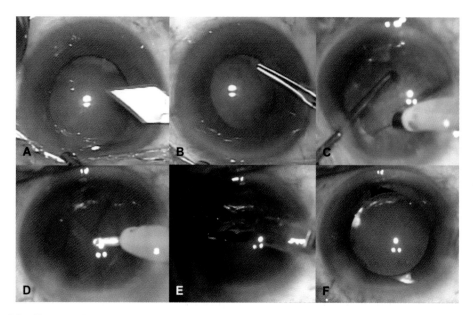

Fig. 3.2. Showing the steps of phacoemulsification including (A) wound creation, (B) capsulorhexis, (C) phacoemulsification of lens material, (D) removal of soft lens material using an irrigation/aspiration probe, (E) implantation of a foldable intraocular lens, and the final image of the (F) completed surgery.

What are the Known Complications of Phacoemulsification?

- Endophthalmitis (potentially blinding complication)
- Posterior capsular rupture
- Dropped nucleus or nuclear fragment
- Suprachoroidal haemorrhage
- Others — raised intraocular pressure from retained viscoelastic, retained lens material, retinal detachment, posterior capsular opacity, bullous keratopathy, sympathetic ophthalmia

What are the Risk Factors for a Complicated Cataract Surgery?

- Poorly cooperative patient
- Small pupil
- Brunescent cataract
- Subluxed cataract
- Presence of zonulysis
- Narrow angles
- Floppy iris
  - Seen in patients on α_{1a} adrenergic antagonist (tamsulosin, prazosin, terazosin, doxazosin)
- Surgeon factor

Take home messages

- Mainstay of treatment for a visually significant cataract is cataract surgery.
- Everyone will eventually develop cataracts, but surgical indication is dependent on various other factors and the individual's visual needs.

References

1. Chylack LT, Jr., Wolfe JK, Singer DM, *et al.* (1993) The Lens Opacities Classification System III. The Longitudinal Study of Cataract Study Group. *Arch Ophthal* (Chicago, Ill : 1960) **111**(6):831–6.

Chapter 4

GLAUCOMA

4.1 Primary Angle Closure Glaucoma

Learning Objectives
- To be able to learn the characteristics of primary angle closure glaucoma and its clinical features.
- To recognise acute angle closure and its immediate management.

What is Primary Angle Closure Glaucoma?
- Subtype of glaucoma characterised by narrow anterior chamber angle and iridotrabecular contact. This can be demonstrated at the slit lamp (Fig. 4.1)

Who is at Risk of Developing Primary Angle Closure Glaucoma?
Risks for PACG are multifactorial
- Systemic risk factors
  - Older age
  - Female gender
  - Ethnicity: East Asian and Inuit
  - Genetics: 3 – 5 times greater risk of developing PACG with positive family history of first-degree relatives

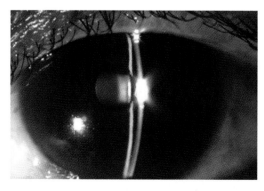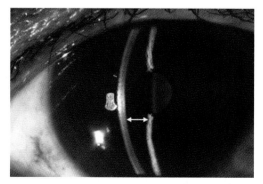

Fig. 4.1. (*Left*) Showing shallow anterior chamber depth and a deeper anterior chamber depth (*Right*). Note the difference in distance between the two light beams (white double-headed arrow) which is used to estimate anterior chamber depth.

- Ocular risk factors
  - Shallow anterior chamber depth
  - Shorter axial length or hyperopia
  - Increased lens vault: Thick lens and/or anteriorly positioned lens

How is the Anterior Chamber Angle Assessed?

- The anterior chamber angle can be assessed either clinically (with gonioscopy) or with anterior segment imaging (e.g. anterior segment optical coherence tomography and ultrasound biomicroscopy). This will be covered in detail in Chapter 4.4.

All patients referred for glaucoma evaluation require a standardised anterior chamber angle assessment.

- Gonioscopy is still the current gold standard

How do you Manage Eyes with Narrow Angles?

- Management needs to be individualised depending on:
  - Aetiology of the angle closure (primary or secondary)
  - Stage of angle closure
  - Mechanism of angle closure
  - Adequacy of the preceding treatment
- The primary aim is to achieve an open angle with an acceptable target IOP with minimal side effects of treatment.
- For primary angle closure suspect, the options include the following:
  - Conservative monitoring with adequate education on symptoms and signs of APAC
  - Laser peripheral iridotomy
    - i. The most common mechanism is pupil block and laser peripheral iridotomy (Fig. 4.2) is an effective prophylaxis against an acute angle closure attack
  - Other considerations for performing laser peripheral iridotomy in patients with PACS include
    - i. Require frequent dilated fundus examination
    - ii. Using drugs that cause pupillary dilation

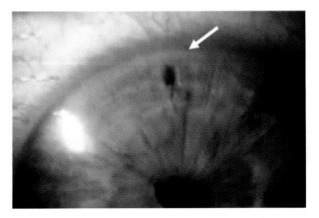

Fig. 4.2. Photograph showing a patent peripheral iridotomy (white arrow).

    iii. Poorly educated patients or patients with reduced awareness who cannot identify symptoms of acute primary angle closure (APAC)

    iv. Patients who are noncompliant or has difficulty accessing ophthalmic care during an APAC episode

- For eyes with angle closure and raised IOP i.e. primary angle closure
  - Perform laser peripheral iridotomy first
  - If target IOP is still not reached, then patient should be started on topical IOP-lowering drugs
- For primary angle closure glaucoma, the patient's IOP should be optimised based on the age, severity of glaucoma and presenting IOP. The target IOP should be reached in a step-wise approach (see Chapter 4.5)
  - Medical therapy
  - Laser
  - Surgical intervention

Clinical Case Study

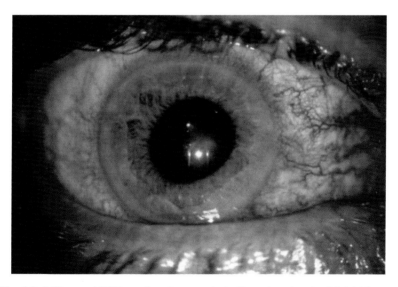

Fig. 4.3. A 70-year-old Chinese female presented with acute red and painful right eye.

What is the Diagnosis? (Fig. 4.3)

- Acute primary angle closure (APAC)

This is a common EOPT question because APAC is an ocular emergency with significant visual morbidity if diagnosis is missed in the primary eye care setting.

Differential Diagnoses

- Acute anterior uveitis
- Endophthalmitis
- Scleritis

What are the Risk Factors of APAC?

The risk factors for APAC can be divided into systemic and ocular

Systemic	Ocular
Older age	Hypermetropia or shorter axial length
Chinese and Inuit race	Shallow anterior chamber depth
Female	Anterior lens vault
Family history of angle closure	Thicker peripheral iris

What are the Symptoms and Signs of APAC?

The typical symptoms of APAC are:
- Acute onset and unilateral
- Eye redness and pain
- Frontal headache
- Nausea and vomiting
- Blurring of vision
- Preceding intermittent glares and haloes

The common signs of APAC include (in order of deceasing importance):

1. **Shallow anterior chamber depth** (note how close the two vertical beams of lights are to each other).	Fig. 4.4 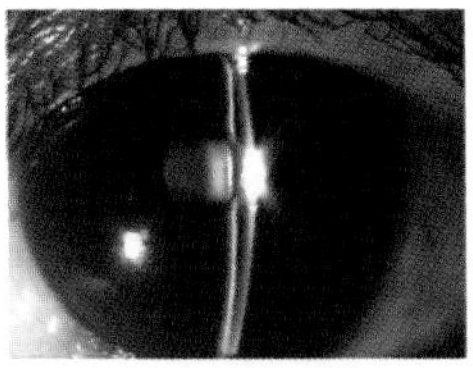	
2. Gonioscopy showing **closed angle in both eyes** (note that the typical angle structures are obscured by anterior bowing of the peripheral iris).	Fig. 4.5 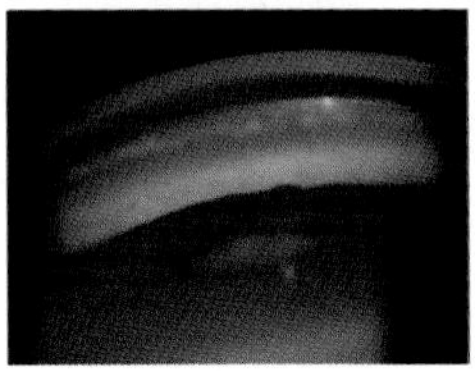	
3. **Raised intraocular pressure** which is measured using the Goldmann applanation tonometry.		
4. **Mid-dilated pupil** which is non-reactive due to iris ischaemia from the raised intraocular pressure.	Fig. 4.6 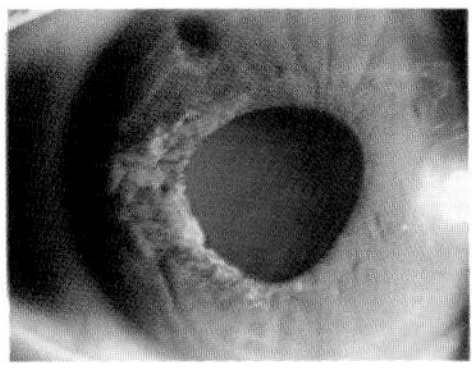	
5. **Conjunctival injection** and **hazy oedematous cornea** due to the high intraocular pressure and ocular inflammation.	Fig. 4.7 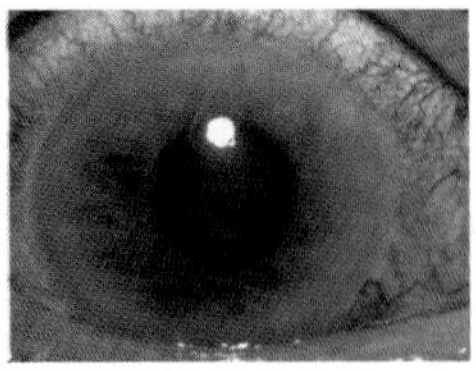	

What is the Immediate Treatment for APAC?

APAC is an ocular emergency which requires urgent treatment to reduce intraocular pressure and relieve the pupil block. The key is prompt diagnosis and referral to the ophthalmologist

The principles of management of APAC are highlighted in the table below:

Principle	Management
1) Reduce IOP promptly	• Fast acting topical IOP-lowering drugs: e.g. brimonidine, timolol • Topical steroids • Topical miotics • Systemic acetazolamide • Peripheral laser iridoplasty • AC paracentesis • Anderson's manoeuvre • Lie supine
2) Eliminate pupil block and non-pupil-block mechanisms	• Laser peripheral iridotomy • Surgical irdectomy • Cataract extraction
3) Assess and treat the fellow eye	• Laser peripheral iridotomy • Other treatment based on mechanisms
4) Monitoring for progression into CACG	• Anterior segment imaging • Visual fields • Optic nerve head imaging

Take home messages

• Anterior chamber angle assessment is important to diagnose angle closure glaucoma.

• The management depends on the mechanism of angle closure, stage of disease and adequacy of preceding treatment.

• Acute angle closure is an ocular emergency. It requires prompt diagnosis and early treatment.

4.2 Primary Open Angle Glaucoma

Learning Objectives

• Learn the definition of primary open angle glaucoma and the investigations required to make an accurate diagnosis.

• Identify the characteristic visual field defects associated with glaucoma.

• Definition of congenital glaucoma and its management principles.

What is Primary Open Angle Glaucoma (POAG)?

POAG is:

• **An irreversible optic neuropathy;** with

• **Characteristic optic disc changes;** and

• **Corresponding visual field defects**

- Commonly but not always associated with raised intraocular pressure

Raised intraocular pressure does NOT equate to POAG.

In POAG, the anterior chamber angles are open for least 270° on gonioscopy without any evidence of iridotrabecular contact. Clinically, there must not be any secondary cause of trabecular outflow obstruction (Fig. 4.8)

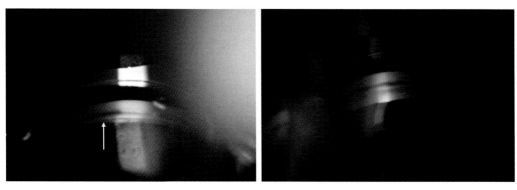

Fig. 4.8. Photographs showing gonioscopic comparison of open angle (Left) and angle closure (Right). In POAG, the angle structures can be visualised especially the posterior trabecular meshwork on gonioscopy (brown pigmented band indicated by white arrow). There is absence of new vessels, peripheral anterior synechiae, pigmentation, blood in Schlemm's canal (signifying raised episcleral venous pressure). In contrast, the image on the right shows angle closure — none of the normal anterior chamber angle structures can be seen.

What are Risk Factors of POAG?

Major	Minor
• Afro-Carribean race • Family history of POAG (2–3x increased risk) • Increased intraocular pressure • Increased age	• Myopia • Hypertension • Diabetes

What are Symptoms of POAG?

- Most commonly asymptomatic due to the chronicity of the disease
- Patients can have headache or eye pain when the intraocular pressure builds up or when the cornea begins to decompensate
- In advanced disease, loss of peripheral vision resulting in "tunnel vision"

What are Optic Nerves Changes Characteristic of POAG?

- Characteristic "hard" signs of the optic nerve
  - Gradual thinning of neurosensory rim starting at the inferior and superior quadrants first (Fig. 4.9)
  - Vertical cup-disc ratio > 0.6
  - Vertical cup-disc ratio asymmetry between eyes > 0.2 (Fig. 4.10)
  - Focal notching of the neuro-retinal rim

- Optic disc drance haemorrhage (Fig. 4.11)
- Retinal nerve fiber layer defect (Fig. 4.12)
- Acquired pit of the optic nerve
- Overhanging optic disc vessels crossing the neuro-retinal rim
- Minor changes
  - 360° of peripapillary atrophy (thinning of retina or RPE around optic nerve)
  - Bayonetting/nasalisation of the blood vessels crossing the optic nerve

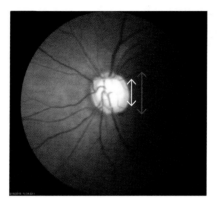

Fig. 4.9. Photograph showing **increased vertical cup-disc ratio** (white arrow = cup height; red arrow = disc height)

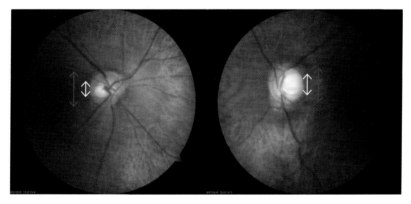

Fig. 4.10. The right and left eye of the same patient showing **vertical cup-disc ratio asymmetry** of more than 0.2 (note: the right image shows the left eye).

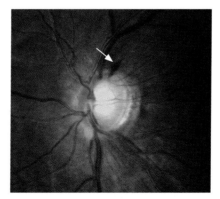

Fig. 4.11. Photograph showing optic disc **drance haemorrhage** (white arrow).

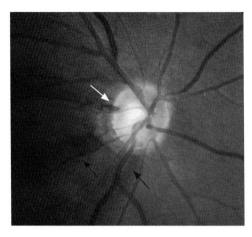

Fig. 4.12. Photograph showing a **wedge inferior retinal nerve fibre defects** (red arrows) and a **drance haemorrhage** of the optic nerve (white arrow).

What are Typical Visual Field Defect Patterns on Automated Perimetry?

- Visual defects associated with glaucoma can be classified into early and late. It can also be classified based on anatomy

- In glaucoma, it is important to note that the visual field defects should correspond to the structural abnormality

  - e.g. A vertical cup-disc ratio of 0.9 can be expected to have a constricted visual field and vice versa. Similarly, an inferior neuroretinal rim notch is associated with a superior visual field defect

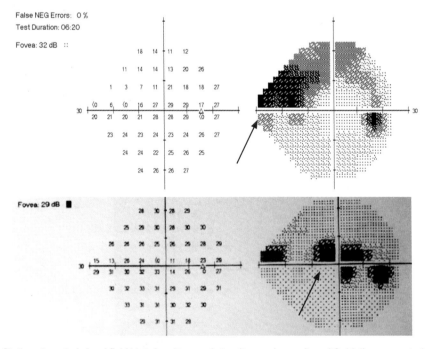

Fig. 4.13. Static automated visual field test showing nasal step (top, red arrow), and Seidel's paracentral scotoma (bottom, blue arrow) of the right eyes of different patients.

- Early visual field loss
  - Nasal step (Fig. 4.13)
  - Seidel's scotoma (Fig. 4.13)
  - Bjerrum scotoma
- Late visual field loss
  - Arcuate visual field loss
  - Constricted visual fields with "tunnel vision"

Clinical Case Study

A 2-month-old baby was referred to the ophthalmologist after the paediatrician notices that there were bilateral cloudy corneas and the baby's eyes appeared "bigger than usual"

What are the Differentials?

- Congenital glaucoma (most important diagnosis to consider)
- Sclerocornea
- Peter's anomaly
- Muchopolysacharidosis

Take home messages
- POAG has a characteristic optic nerve appearance with corresponding visual field defect.
- Raised intraocular pressure is only a risk factor for POAG.
- Apart from a raised cup-disc ratio, there are other optic nerve features of POAG.

4.3 Secondary Glaucoma

Learning Objectives
- Identify the different types and mechanisms of secondary glaucoma.
- Outline the main principles of management specific to the aetiology of secondary glaucoma.

What are the Types of Secondary Glaucoma?

- Open angle
  - Causes can be divided into pre-trabecular meshwork (TM), trabecular meshwork and post-trabecular meshwork
    - i. Pre-TM: ICE syndrome (Fig. 4.14), epithelial downgrowth, tumours, aphakia
    - ii. TM: Hyphema, inflammatory (uveitis, tumours), NVG, pigments, PXF, steroids, iatrogenic (silicone oil)
    - iii. Post-TM: Carotid-cavernous tistula, Sturge Weber syndrome
- Angle closure
  - Causes can be divided into push and pull mechanisms
    - i. Push: lens-induced, lens subuxation, ciliary body cysts/tumours, iatrogenic (SO or scleral buckle), aqueous misdirection/drugs (topiramate, sulfonamide, anti-cholinergics)
    - ii. Pull: AAU, NVG, ICE, aniridia

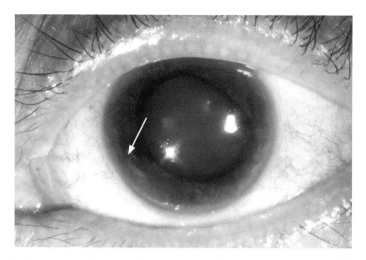

Fig. 4.14. Showing high peripheral anterior synechiae (white arrow) characteristic of ICE syndrome.

What is Traumatic Glaucoma?

Subtype of secondary glaucoma due to significant ocular trauma resulting in either open or closed angle obstruction of aqueous outflow from the eye

What are the Mechanisms of Traumatic Glaucoma?

Open Angle	Angle Closure
• Angle recession glaucoma (Fig. 4.15)	• Subluxed lens
• Steroid-induced glaucoma	• Dense cataracts
• Hyphema (risk of re-bleeding is highest around 3–5 days after injury; higher risk if hyphema is more than 1/3 of AC depth, sickle cell disease, or on anti-coagulation drugs) (Fig. 4.16)	• Peripheral anterior synechiae (PAS)
• Ghost cell glaucoma	

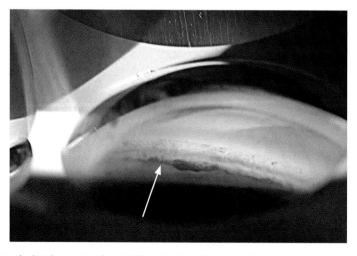

Fig. 4.15. Photograph showing a **prominent ciliary body** (white arrow) in angle recession syndrome after trauma.

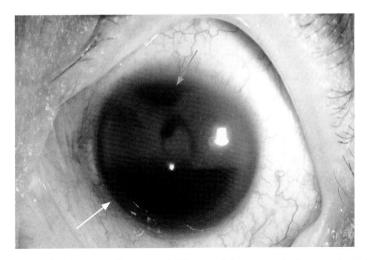

Fig. 4.16. Photograph showing **gross hyphema** (white arrow) from **superior haemorrhage** (blue arrow).

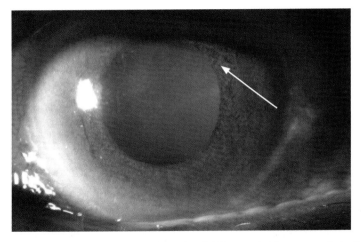

Fig. 4.17. Photograph showing florid iris neovascularisation (white arrow). Iris neovascularisation is usually the most prominent around pupillary borders.

What are the Causes of Neovascular Glaucoma (NVG)?

- Most common causes of NVG (Fig. 4.17) are:
  - Proliferative diabetic retinopathy
  - Ischaemic central vein occlusion
  - Ocular ischaemic syndrome
- Less common causes include:
  - Chronic retinal detachment
  - Chronic uveitis (e.g. VKH, Behcet's disease)
  - Ocular tumours (e.g. choroidal melanoma, retinoblastoma)
  - Carotid-cavernous fistula
  - Ocular tumours (e.g. choroidal melanoma, retinoblastoma)
  - Carotid-cavernous fistula

How is NVG Treated?

NVG is a difficult condition to treat and the visual prognosis is guarded. The subsequent management depends on the underlying cause, visual prognosis and patient symptoms

- Reduce intraocular pressure and relieve pain
  - Topical and systemic drugs to lower intraocular pressure
  - Topical cycloplegics
  - Intravitreal injection of anti-vascular endothelial growth factor
- Determine the cause and reduce ischaemic drive
  - Perform panretinal laser photocoagulation if no media opacity
- Subsequent intraocular pressure control depends on visual prognosis
  - Good visual prognosis: glaucoma shunt surgery
  - Poor visual prognosis:
    - i. Painful: trans-scleral cyclophotocoagulation
      - If blind, consider evisceration
    - ii. Painless: conservative
      - Topical IOP-lowering medications
      - Topical cycloplegics

Clinical Case Study

A 30-year-old African American female with a history of sarcoidosis presented with right eye redness and blurring of vision for 1 week. Examination showed anterior chamber cells and granulomatous keratic precipitates (Fig. 4.18). Her intraocular pressure is 35 mmHg in the right eye

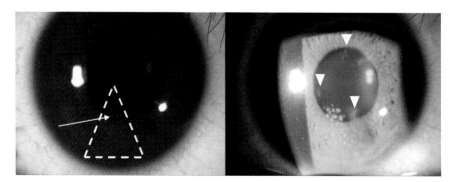

Fig. 4.18. (Left) Shows granulomatous keratic precipiatates (white arrow) on inferior corneal endothelium forming the Arlt's triangle (dotted triangle). (Right) Shows the same eye with posterior synechiae which is adhesion between the iris and anterior lens surface (arrowheads). The keratic precipitates are once again visualised.

What are the Mechanisms of Raised Intraocular Pressure in this lady?

Open Angle	Angle Closure
• Angle failure due to chronic and recurrent inflammation	• Peripheral anterior synaechiae
• Steroid-induced	• Extensive posterior synaechiae causing seclusio pupillae
• Neovascularisation	

What are the Causes of Hypertensive Uveitis?

Infective	Non-infective
• Viral: CMV, HSV, VZV, rubella	• Matsuo-Schwatz from retinal detachment
• Bacterial: bacterial endophthalmitis, syphilis, toxoplamosis	• Sarcoidosis

Clinical Case Study

A 79-year-old man with pre-existing poor vision in the right eye was punched in the same eye during a domestic dispute. He presented with right eye pain, redness, nausea and vomiting 2 days after the incident. On examination, you find the following (Fig. 4.19):

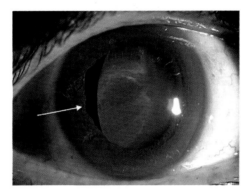

Fig. 4.19. Photograph of the patient's right eye showing infero-temporal subluxation of a cataractous lens. The zonular fibres are not well visualised, and the iris margins are irregular nasally (white arrow), suggesting possible sphincter rupture.

What has Happened to the Right Eye of this patient?

He has a dense cataract which has also subluxed inferiorly

What are the Types of Lens-induced Glaucoma?

Angle Closure	Open Angle
• Subluxed lens • Dense cataract causing **phacomorphic** glaucoma	• **Phacoanaphylactic**: breached lens capsule with result leak of lens material inciting AC inflammation • **Phacolytic**: intact anterior lens capsule through which lens material leak causing AC inflammation

What are some Risk Factors for Lens Subluxation?

Congenital	Acquired
• Ectopia lentis • Connective tissue disease: Marfan, Ehler-Danlos, Homocysteinuria	• Ocular trauma • Dense brunescent cataract • Myopia • Pseudoexfoliation / pigment dispersion syndrome • Tumours (e.g. retinoblastoma, ciliary body melanoma)

Take home messages

- Secondary glaucoma can be sub-divided into open angle and angle closure.
- Neovascular glaucoma is a difficult condition to treat and management depends on aetiology, visual prognosis and symptoms.

4.4 Investigations related to Glaucoma

Learning Objectives

- Familiarise with the common investigations performed for glaucoma patients.
- Learn how to interpret static automated perimetry in a systematic approach.

What are the Investigations Commonly Performed for Glaucoma patients?

- Structural tests
  - Anterior segment
    - i. Anterior segment optical coherence tomography
    - ii. Ultrasound biomicroscopy
    - iii. Photo-gonioscopy
  - Posterior segment
    - i. Stereodisc photographs
    - ii. Confocal laser scanning ophthalmoscopy
    - iii. Optical coherence tomography
- Functional tests
  - Static automated perimetry

What are the Ways to Evaluate Anterior Chamber Angles?

The evaluation of the anterior chamber angles is important in determining the pathogenesis of glaucoma — open or angle closure. There are various modes including:

- Slit lamp gonioscopy
  - Still the **current gold standard**
  - Performed in dark conditions at the slit lamp and using a gonioscope
  - Light from the anterior chamber undergoes total internal reflection and so a contact lens is required to overcome this principle
    - i. The goniolens has a similar refractive index as the cornea and alters the cornea–air interface to overcome the critical angle that prevents total internal refraction of light from the angles
  - Gonioscope lenses can be direct or indirect
    - i. Direct gonioscope is usually used during angle surgery (e.g. goniotomy)
    - ii. Indirect gonioscope can be divided into indentational and non-indentational
      - Indentation is important to differential apposition and synechial angle closure

- **Apposition** refers to contact between the peripheral iris and trabecular meshwork which is reversible
- **Synechial closure** refers to adherent contact between the same structures
- Anterior segment optical coherence tomography (AS-OCT)
  - Provides high resolution cross sectional images of the anterior segment of the eye (Fig. 4.20)
  - Provides qualitative and quantitative assessment of the anterior chamber angles, mechanism of angle closure, lens position and even cornea pathology
- Ultrasound biomicroscopy (UBM)
  - Uses 35–100 MHz frequency transducer which provides resolution up to 25 μm
  - It has better tissue penetration compared to AS-OCT which allows evaluation of structures behind the iris (e.g. ciliary body, pars plana, zonules)

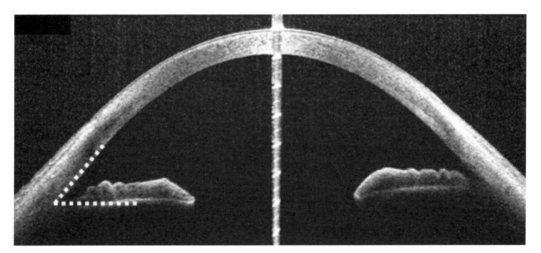

Fig. 4.20A. AS-OCT image showing open angle (white dotted lines).

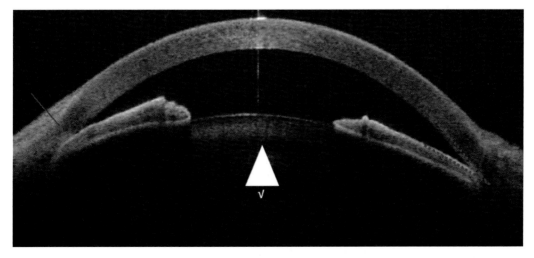

Fig. 4.20B. AS-OCT image showing narrow angles (red dotted lines) with closure in one quadrant (red arrow). The anterior lens vault from cataract is also seen (white arrowhead).

Table Summarising the Advantages and Disadvantages of Various Anterior Chamber Angle Imaging Modalities

	Advantages	Disadvantages
Gonioscopy	• Low cost • Less equipment required • Colour visualisation of the angles (e.g. tumours, FB, NVA) • Can indent to differentiate appositional vs synechial angle closure	• Poor reproducibility • Not quantifiable • Operator dependent • Cannot visualise behind iris
AS-OCT	• Non-contact • Fast • Reproducible • Latest Swept-Source OCT allows 360° assessment of the angles • Quantifiable parameters	• Cannot visualise behind the iris • Expensive
UBM	• Cannot visualise behind the iris	• Operator dependent • Only in supine position • Time-consuming • Expensive

Why is Structural Imaging of the Optic Nerve Head Important and How is it done?

Histologic and imaging studies have shown that structural changes to the optic nerve head or retinal nerve fibre layer precedes functional changes – up to 40% of retinal ganglion cell loss may have occurred before any detectable visual field loss appears

Common imaging modalities used in the clinical setting:

- Stereodisc photographs
  - The earliest form of optic nerve imaging
- Optical coherence tomography (e.g. Cirrus® OCT-RNFL)
  - Uses low coherence laser interferometry to acquire high resolution cross-sectional images of the eye
    - i. Current spectral domain OCT can collect up to 55,000 A-scans per second with a resolution of 5μm
  - Measures parameters of the optic nerve head, retinal nerve fibre layer and the macular ganglion cell layer
- Confocal scanning laser ophthalmoscopy (e.g. HRT)
  - Uses a diode laser of wavelength 670 nm as light source
  - Takes multiple images (maximum of 64 slices) of the optic nerve from superficial to deep layers then combine all the images to recreate 3-D reconstruction of the optic nerve head
  - Provides both area and volumetric measurements of the optic nerve head
- Scanning laser polarimetry (e.g. GDx-VCC)
  - Use of polarised light to measure thickness of the retinal nerve fibre layer
  - Seldom used nowadays

Table Summarising the Advantages and Disadvantages of Various Optic Nerve Head Structural Imaging Modalities

	Advantages	Disadvantages
Stereodisc (Fig. 4.21)	• Affordable • Colour images can show disc haemorrhages or disc pallor • Not affected by change in technology upgrades	• Cannot detect small changes in optic nerve head, making monitoring difficult • Only 2-dimensional: only certain structural defects (e.g. cup-disc ratio and disc size are seen)
OCT (Fig. 4.22)	• Non-contact • Fast • Highly-reproducible • Guided progression analysis to detect structural progression using retinal nerve fibre layer thickness	• Expensive • Floor effect: for advanced disease, OCT measurements level off and does not fall below $50 - 70\,\mu m$ • Media opacity can affect signal quality • Normative database does not include eyes with high myopia
HRT	• Optic nerve head visualisation • Long track record • Fast and reproducible • Progression analysis programme — topographic change analysis	• Does not provide reliable retinal nerve fibre layer measurements • Lack of a large ethnic-specific normative database • Optic nerve head parameters significantly affected by different morphology, e.g. optic disc tilt • Manual delineation of optic disc margin required by observe
GDx	• Seldom used nowadays	

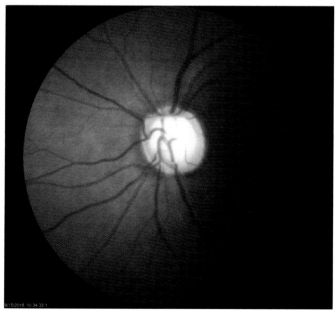

Fig. 4.21. Disc photograph showing increased cup-disc ratio. Colour disc photographs are useful as an objective documentation of disc appearance as a baseline.

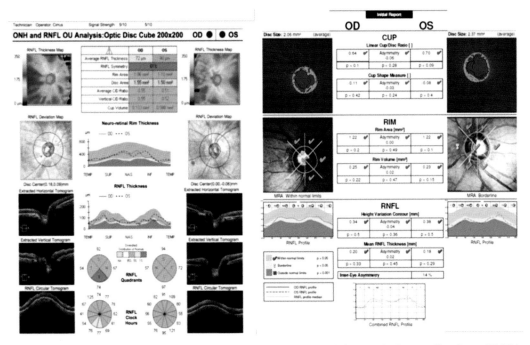

Fig. 4.22. Left image showing a typical **OCT** printout, demonstrating inferior retinal nerve fibre layer (RNFL) thinning in the right eye (red quadrant inferiorly). Right)image shows a typical HRT printout.

Clinical Case Study

A 50-year-old Chinese female with a family history of glaucoma wants to check her risk of glaucoma. The following test (Fig. 4.23) was performed in the clinic:

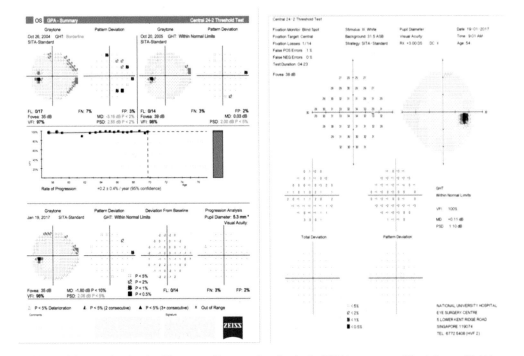

Fig. 4.23. Left image showing the **Glaucoma Progression Analysis (GPA)** summary of the left eye. Right image shows a typical printout of the **Humphrey visual field** test.

What is the Test being Shown below?

- Static automated perimetry testing the central 24° of fixation using the SITA standard algorithm
- Perimetry refers to the measurement of one's visual field — defined as the space that one eye can see while maintaining fixation at a single target

What Testing Strategies are Available?

Suprathreshold	Full Threshold	SITA
• Rapid screening test • Light stimulus is very intense and is the same across the whole visual field • Output is categorical – "Yes" or "No" only	• Retinal sensitivity is tested at each point using bracketing method • Time consuming but provides point-by-point qualitative data • Duration of test can be shortened using artificial interlligence such as the Swedish Interactive Threshold Algorithm (SITA)	• Based on Bayesian probability and estimates the retinal sensitivity as each point • Uses real time calculation to estimate adjacent threshold values based on pateint's individual response • Preferred by clinicians due to the shorter test duration without affecting diagnostic performance

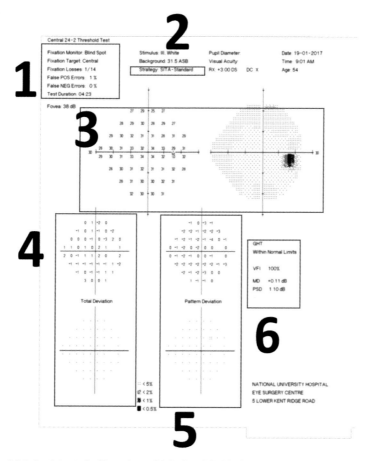

Fig. 4.24. A printout of a **Humphrey 24-2 visual field** of a normal patient's right eye.

How to Interpret the Static Automated Perimetry Results (Fig. 4.24)**?**

1. Determine the boundary of visual field testing (common: central 24, 30 or 10 degrees) and the reliability of the test (see below)

2. Check the test strategies used and whether they are consistent with previous tests especially when monitoring for progression

3. Raw values plots provide the raw threshold values of each point for the individual patient

4. Total deviation plots refers to the deviation of each individual test point compared to the age-matched normal controls

5. Pattern deviation plots adjust for generalised reduction in retinal sensitivity (due to refractive errors or cataracts) and reveal the underlying localised visual field defects or scotomas

6. Global indices: these secondary summary values are derived from the raw data and provide the clinician with an overall impression of the results

- Glaucoma Hemifield Test (GHT)
  - Compares 5 zones in the superior and corresponding 5 zones in the inferior hemifield. The extent of asymmetry is used as an indicator for glaucoma. The possible results are: within normal limits, outside normal limits and borderline

- Visual field index (VFI)
  - Expresses visual field status as a % of a normal age-matched visual field
  - Greater weight is given to points closer to fixation to adjust for differential ganglion cell density
  - Less affected by cataracts or after cataract surgery
  - Commonly used as a marker to track visual progression

- Mean deviation (MD)
  - Average deviation of each point from age-matched normal controls
  - In general more minus is bad (**M** for MD)

- Pattern standard deviation (PSD)
  - Indicator the variability of all the points within the visual fields
  - In general more plus is bad (**P** for PSD)

How do you Evaluate the Reliability of this test?

- The static automated perimetry is a subjective test and has 3 main reliability indices
  - Fixation loss: a surrogate measure of how well the patient keeps fixation at a fixed target in primary gaze. In general, a fixation loss of less than 20% is acceptable
  - False positive: a high value indicates a "trigger-happy" patient who responds even though he/she did not detect any light stimulation. A value of less than 30% is acceptable
  - False negative: a high value suggests an "inattentive" patient who did not respond to a repeated stimulation which he/she has responded to earlier in the test. A value of less than 30% is acceptable
  - Other tests of reliability includes the eyelid movement and eye movement tracker

How can Static Perimetry be Monitored in a patient with Glaucoma?

Serial visual fields can be monitored manually or using automated software. The latter can be broadly classified into:

- Event-based progression analysis
  - Glaucoma progression analysis (GPA) was the first event-based change analysis software to be put into widespread clinical use
  - Identifies significant point-wise progression based on statistical probabilities
  - Requires at least three sequential visual fields
  - Does not require as many fields to detect progression compared to trend-based analysis
- Trend-based progression analysis
  - For clinical practice, this is more practical
  - Allows the clinician to determine the rate of progression/deterioration in visual fields
    i. Provides extrapolated data based on trend analysis
    ii. Uses either the visual field index or mean deviation as the summary measure of the global retinal sensitivity

---

Take home messages

- Gonioscopy is still the gold standard for anterior chamber angle evaluation but the anterior segment optical coherence tomography and ultrasound biomicroscopy imaging are alternatives.
- Structural imaging of the optic nerve head provides an objective measurement for monitoring purpose.
- Static automated perimetry is a subjective test and the reliability indices need to be assessed prior to interpretation.

4.5 Management of Glaucoma and its Complications

Learning Objectives

- Learn the principles and indications for medical, laser and surgical therapy for glaucoma.
- Identify the potential side effects or complications associated with therapy.

What do you Understand by Target Intraocular Pressure (IOP)?

Target IOP needs to be individualised and is the IOP level (or below) in which functional and structural progression of glaucoma is prevented. Target IOP depends on the age/life expectancy, presenting IOP and severity of glaucoma

How can a Target IOP Be Achieved?

- Medical
  - Aqueous suppressants
    i. **A**lpha agonist: Brimonidine (Alphagan®)
    ii. **B**eta blocker: Timolol
    iii. **C**arbonic anhydrase inhibitor (both topical and systemic): Acetazolamide (Azopt®), Dorzolamide (Trusopt®)

- Increase aqueous outflow
    - i. Alpha agonist
    - ii. **P**rostaglandin analogue: Latanoprost (Xalatan®), Bimatoprost (Lumigan®)
    - iii. **P**ilocarpine
- Hyperosmotic agents
    - i. Mannitol
    - ii. Glycerine
- Fixed combination drugs
    - i. Usually in combination with a beta-blocker
    - ii. Improve compliance to medications by rationalising daily regime

- Lasers
    - Iris
        - i. Laser peripheral iridotomy
            - Relieves pupil block and widen anterior chamber angle
            - Key treatment for acute angle closure
        - ii. Laser peripheral iridoplasty (Fig. 4.26)
            - Treats plateau iris syndrome
            - Can be used to temporarily reduce IOP in acute angle closure
    - Trabecular meshwork
        - i. Selective laser trabeculoplasty
            - Effective for primary open angle glaucoma and pigmentary glaucoma
            - Effect may be temporary and suitable for following patients
                - Unfit for surgery
                - Not keen for surgery
                - Pregnancy
            - Increases aqueous outflow through the trabecular meshwork due to both mechanical and biochemical mediators
        - ii. Ciliary body
            - Cyclophotocoagulation
                - Reduces aqueous production by reducing ciliary body volume
                - Can be delivered trans-scleral or endoscopically
                - Typically reserved for refractory glaucoma with poor visual prognosis
                - Risk of pthisis bulbi and sympathetic ophthalmia
                - Micropulse mode is increasingly popular
                    - More gentle to the ciliary body compared to traditional TCP
                    - Can be repeated multiple times if necessary
                    - Lower risk of pthsis bulbi

- Surgery
  - Main indication for surgical intervention is the presence of functional or structural deterioration and inability to achieve target IOP despite maximum tolerable medical therapy
  - Aim is to improve aqueous drainage by maximising innate outflow facility or create an alternative outflow path
  - Phacoemulsification
    - i. Indicated for angle closure eyes in which the "bulky" lens (usually also has significant cataract) contributes to angle narrowing
    - ii. Removal of cataract and replacement with a thinner intraocular lens improves the trabecular meshwork drainage of aqueous and lowers IOP
    - iii. Can be combined with goniosynechiolysis to release early peripheral anterior synechiae
    - iv. In eyes with mild glaucoma, phacoemulsification can be augmented with minimally invasive glaucoma surgery devices to increase aqueous outflow to the schlemm canal, subconjunctival space or suprachoroidal space
  - Trabeculectomy (Fig. 4.25)
    - i. A guarded fistula between the anterior chamber and the subconjunctival space through a sclerostomy and a partial thickness scleral flap
    - ii. Still the most popular first-line surgical intervention
  - Aqueous shunts (Fig. 4.26)
    - i. Reserved for eyes at high risk of trabeculectomy failure or previous failed trabeculectomy
    - ii. Involves the use of a silicone tube shunting aqueous from the anterior chamber to the post-equatorial subconjunctival space
    - iii. The conjunctiva at the equator has less fibroblast and less exposed to the external environment making it less likely to scar down
    - iv. Classified into valved and non-valve implants
      - Valved implant
        - Built-in valve within the tube regulates aqueous flow and could prevent post-operative hypotony
        - For example, Ahmed glaucoma implant, Krupin implant
      - Non-valved implant
        - The lack of any flow regulator means these implants require supplemental constriction of the tube caliber using restorable sutures. These sutures can be removed subsequently when conjunctival healing around the base plate is deemed adequate.
        - However, the risk of hypotony is higher for this group of implants
        - For example, Baerveldt implant, Molteno implant

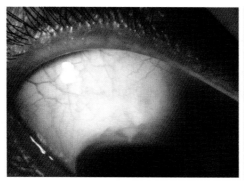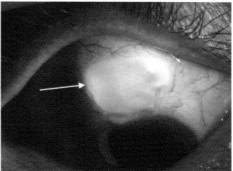

Fig. 4.25. Left image shows a diffuse and healthy trabeculectomy bleb. Right image shows a cystic, thin and avascular bleb (white arrow); this bleb is more prone to complications and failure.

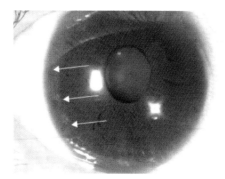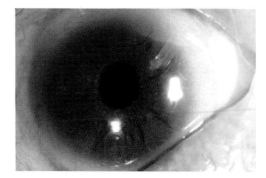

Fig. 4.26. Left image shows **iridoplasty scars** (white arrows). Right image shows a well-placed **Ahmed tube** (red arrow).

What are the Potential Side Effects of IOP-lowering Medications?

	Ocular	Systemic
Beta-blockers	• Reduced corneal sensation	• Bronchospasm • Bradycardia • Masks hypoglycemic effect in diabetics • Lethargy • Decreased libido
Alpha-agonists	• Conjunctival hyperemia • Allergic conjunctivitis • Reactivation of HSV keratitis	• Central nervous system depression in children (crosses the immature blood-brain barrier)
Carbonic anhydrase inhibitor	• Reduced endothelial pump function	• Allergy/anaphylaxia • Stevens-Johnson syndrome • Metabolic acidosis • Renal stones • Reduced appetite and metallic taste • Tingling sensation on fingertips and toes

Prostaglandin analogue	• Conjunctival hyperaemia	• Minimal
	• Allergic conjunctivitis	
	• Hypertrichosis	
	• Hyperpigmentation of iris and periocular tissue	
	• Periorbital fat atrophy	
	• Cystoid macular oedema	
	• Pro-inflammatory and breaks down blood-aqueous barrier (relative contraindication for uveitis)	

What are Risks and Complications of Trabeculectomy?

- Intraoperative
  - Suprachoroidal haemorrhage
  - Conjunctival button-hole
- Early post-operative
  - Shallow AC
    i. High IOP
    - Suprachoroidal haemorrhage
    - Pupil block
    - Malignant glaucoma/Aqueous misdirection
    ii. Low IOP
    - Overfiltration
    - Conjunctiva leak
  - Hyphaema
  - Endophthalmitis
  - Wipe-out
    i. Loss of remaining vision due to advanced visual field loss
- Late postoperative
  - High IOP due to subconjunctival fibrosis
  - Chronic hypotony
    i. From bleb leak
    ii. From cystic avascular bleb
  - Blebitis and endophthalmitis
  - Cataract progression

What are Risk Factors for Trabeculectomy Failure?

Patient Factors	Ocular Factors
• Young patient	• Secondary glaucoma
• Asian, African-Americans	• Chronic use of IOP-lowering eye drops
• Prone to scarring (e.g. keloid formation)	• Previous failed trabeculectomy

What are the Indications for Laser Iridotomy?

- Main objective for laser iridotomy is to relieve pupil block
  - Most common mechanism for angle closure
- Pupil block results from relative resistance between the lens and pupillary margin
  - Results in differential pressure between the posterior and anterior chamber
  - Classic iris bombe configuration
  - Forward bowing of the iris results in contact between the trabecular meshwork and peripheral iris
  - Occlusion of the anterior chamber angles prevents aqueous drainage and results in a build-up of intraocular pressure
- Laser iridotomy neutralises the differential pressure gradient anterior and posterior to the iris resulting in iris flattening
- As such, laser iridotomy is performed for eyes with
  - Occludable angles
  - Primary or secondary angle closure glaucoma
  - Acute primary angle closure

What are the Complications associated with Laser Iridotomy?

- Photopsia
  - Due to light entering the eye through the iridotomy site
  - More common if the iridotomy site is near the upper eyelid resting position
- Corneal decompensation
  - Associated with loss of endothelial cell loss
  - Higher risk if there is chronic or acute rise in intraocular pressure
- Hyphema
  - Risk of hyphaema can be reduced by performing sequential argon-YAG laser
  - Argon laser has photocoagulation properties and helps to coagulate blood vessels on the iris as the iris thins out
  - YAG laser aids to widen the iridotomy
- Intraocular pressure spike
- Malignant glaucoma

What are the Complications associated with Aqueous Shunt Surgery?

The complications can be divided into:
- Intraoperative
  - Suprachoroidal haemorrhage
  - Conjunctiva button-hole
  - Hyphema
- Early postoperative
  - Shallow anterior chamber from overfiltration
  - Low IOP
  - Hyphema

i. Usually self-limiting

ii. Blood can block the tube causing raised intraocular pressure

- Late postoperative
  - Cornea decompensation
    - i. Due to tube-cornea touch, persistent iritis, anterior chamber fluctuation
  - Hypertensive phase
    - i. Due to conjunctiva healing and fibrosis
    - ii. Happens between 2 – 6 weeks after surgery
  - Conjunctiva erosion and exposure of tube / plate
  - Diplopia
  - Bleb encapsulation resulting in surgical failure
  - Cataract progression

What are the Symptoms and Signs of Blebitis/Endophthalmitis? How do you Manage them?

Blebitis and / or endophthalmitis (Fig. 4.27) are an ocular emergency because it can progress rapidly and lead to blindness.

Symptoms	Signs

• Red and painful eye
• Reduced vision
	• Swollen periocular tissue
	• Corneal oedema
	• Anterior chamber inflammation including hypopyon
	• Leaking bleb
	  • Bleb may be thin, avascular and cystic
	  • Bleb contents are opaque and filled with fibrin/pus
	• Conjunctiva surrounding the bleb is congested
	• If endophthalmitis is present
	  • Presence of relative afferent pupillary defect
	  • Loss of red reflex
	  • Presence of vitritis

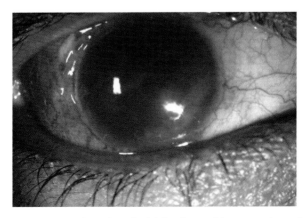

Fig. 4.27. Photograph showing **sectoral conjunctival injection** and **hyperaemia**, and opacification related to blebitis in this patient. Note the corneal oedema and consequent loss of iris details.

What are Risks Factors for Blebitis/Endophthlamitis?

The risk factors for blebitis/endophthalmitis are:

Systemic	Ocular
• Immunocompromised (e.g. renal transplant, elderly, diabetes mellitus)	• Poor ocular surface • Lid disorders (e.g. Meibomian gland dysfunction, blepharitis, trichiasis) • Use of antimetabolites during trabeculectomy • Repeated bleb needling with anti-metabolites

How do you Manage Blebitis or Bleb-related Endophthalmitis?

Principles of management include:

• Microbiological diagnosis

- Conjunctival swab around the bleb
- Vitreous tap if endophthalmitis suspected and inject intravitreal antibiotics in the same setting

• Identify risk factors and treat (e.g. optimise diabetes control, treat blepharitis)

• Anti-microbial therapy

- Empirical treatment with broad spectrum topical antibiotics
- If endophthalmitis suspected, treat with intravitreal antibiotics and systemic antibiotics
- Subsequent anti-microbial regime depends on organism sensitivity

• Repair of bleb

- Once active infection is treated, the trabeculectomy bleb at risk needs to be addressed
- Bleb exploration and repair may be required
- If not possible, compromised bleb needs to be excised and a separate filtration surgery at another site performed

Take home messages

- The target intraocular pressure can be achieved by either increasing aqueous outflow or reducing aqueous production.
- Laser iridotomy is indicated for angle closure to increase anterior chamber angle width.
- The indication for surgical intervention is the presence of functional or structural deterioration and inability to achieve target IOP despite maximum tolerable medical therapy.

References

1. American Academy of Ophthalmology — *Glaucoma*.
2. Shibal Bhartiya — *Manual of Glaucoma*.
3. Tarek M Shaarawy — *Glaucoma*.

Chapter 5

UVEITIS

5.1 Classification

Learning Objectives
• Understanding the definition and classification of uveitis.
• Understanding the descriptors and terminologies used in uveitis.

Classification of Uveitis

Uveitis is defined as inflammation of the uveal tract. The uveal tract comprises the iris, ciliary body and choroid. Various classifications and grading systems for uveitis are available.

• Anatomical
• Clinical
• Aetiological
• Pathological

Definitions

Anterior uveitis

• Iritis: inflammation confined to the anterior chamber.
• Iridocyclitis: inflammation involving the ciliary body is termed as cyclitis. In iridocyclitis, cells are also seen in the retrolental (behind the crystalline lens) space.
• Keratouveitis: inflammation involving the cornea and uveal tract.
• Sclerouveitis: inflammation involving the sclera and uveal tract.

Intermediate uveitis

• Inflammation primarily involving the middle portion of the eye, namely the posterior ciliary body and pars plana
• Inflammatory cells are seen in the vitreous

Posterior uveitis

• Inflammatory cells may be seen diffusely in the vitreous cavity, over the foci of active inflammation, on the posterior vitreous face or they can be absent (e.g. in immunodeficient patients)
• Inflammation can also affect the blood vessels resulting in vasculitis

Panuveitis

- Diffuse inflammation involving the anterior and posterior segment

Anatomical Classification

The Standardisation of Uveitis Nomenclature (SUN) Working Group (2005) amended the anatomical classification that is commonly used today

Table 5.1. The SUN Working Group Anatomical Classification of Uveitis

Type	Primary Site of Inflammation	Includes
Anterior uveitis	Anterior chamber	Anterior chamber
Intermediate uveitis	Vitreous	Vitreous
Posterior uveitis	Retina or choroid	Retina or choroid
Panuveitis	Anterior chamber, vitreous, and retina or choroid	Anterior chamber, vitreous, and retina or choroid

The SUN working group also provided descriptors of uveitis based on the following features

Table 5.2. The SUN Working Group Descriptors of Uveitis

Category	Descriptor	Comment
Onset	Sudden Insidious	
Duration	Limited	< 3 months' duration
	Persistent	≥ 3 months' duration
Course	Acute	Episode characterised by sudden onset and limited duration
	Recurrent	Repeated episodes separated by periods of inactivity without treatment ≥ 3 months duration
	Chronic	Persistent uveitis with relapse in < 3 months after discontinuing treatment

Clinical Classification

The clinical classification is formalised by the International Uveitis Study Group (IUGS)

Table 5.3. The IUSG Clinical Classification of Uveitis

Group	Subgroup
Infectious	Bacterial Viral Fungal Parasitic Others
Non-infectious	Known systemic association No known systemic association
Masquerade	Neoplastic (e.g. lymphoma, leukaemia) Non-neoplastic (e.g. TB)

Aetiological Classification

The aetiological classification expands on the cause of the disease and the treatment options. Nevertheless, often in uveitis, the true underlying aetiology is not known

Pathological Classification

The pathological classification separates granulomatous from non-granulomatous uveitis. Granulomatous uveitis is characterised by large "mutton-fat" keratic precipitates (KPs) formed by macrophages and iris nodules, which include Busacca (located within the iris stroma) and Koeppe (located at the pupillary border) nodules

Take home messages
- Uveitis encompasses a complex set of inflammatory pathologies in the eye.
- Understanding the classification of uveitis will aid in establishing the underlying aetiology and subsequent management.

5.2. Clinical Assessment and Investigations

Clinical Assessment

Learning Objectives
- Learning the approach to assessing a patient with uveitis.
- Learning when to investigate a patient with uveitis.
- Learning the roles of investigation in aiding management of a patient with uveitis.

A thorough ophthalmic history and systematic review followed by detailed examination are paramount in all patients with uveitis.
In certain cases, systemic examination and co-management with an internal physician may be required.

Table 5.4. Ophthalmic History

Symptoms	Dependent on which segment of the uveal tract is inflamed • Anterior: redness, pain, photophobia and blurring of vision • Intermediate: blurring of vision, floaters, photopsia, photophobia • Posterior: typically painless blurring of vision, floaters, scotoma
Past ocular history	Previous similar episode: ask if any investigations were performed, results of investigations, any treatment? Previous history of ocular trauma or surgery (think of sympathetic ophthalmia)
Past medical history	• Systemic inflammatory disorders (e.g. sarcoidosis, Behcet's disease) • HLA-B27 associated spondyloarthropathies, rheumatoid arthritis • Chronic infection (e.g. TB, syphilis, HSV) • Immunocompromised status (e.g. malignancy, post-transplant, intravenous drug user)

Family history	Family history of uveitis or systemic inflammatory disorders
Drug history	Systemic immunosuppression and medications
Occupational history	

Table 5.5. Ophthalmic Examination

Visual function	Presenting visual acuity Relative afferent pupillary defect (RAPD), colour vision
Signs of uveitis (anterior) on slit-lamp examination	Conjunctiva • Perilimbal (Fig. 5.1) or diffuse injection Cornea • Keratic precipitates (Fig. 5.2) Anterior chamber: • Cells • Flare (proteinaceous influx) • Fibrin (Fig. 5.3) • Hypopyon Iris • Nodules • Anterior or posterior synechiae • Atrophy • Heterochromia Intraocular pressure • Hypotony • Secondary glaucoma – open or closed angle
Signs of uveitis (posterior) on slit-lamp examination with condensing lens (e.g. 90D for better evaluation of vitreous cells, 78D for better assessment of macular details)	Vitreous • Cells (single or clumped), snowballs • Tractional bands Pars plana • Snowbanking Retina • Unifocal or multifocal retinitis (fluffy white lesions which may progress to necrosis, atrophy which may lead to retinal detachment in the presence of atrophic retinal holes) • Cystoid macular oedema • Serous retinal detachment • Epiretinal membrane • Vasculitis Choroid • Unifocal or multifocal choroiditis (blurred yellowish lesions deep to the retina)

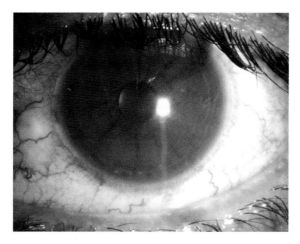

Fig. 5.1. Perilimbal injection.

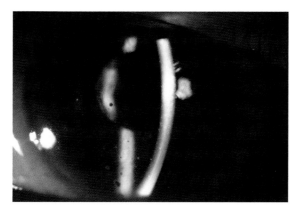

Fig. 5.2. Mutton-fat keratic precipitate in granulomatous uveitis.

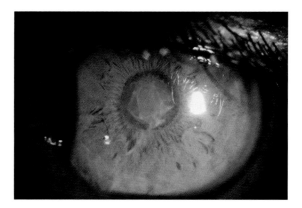

Fig. 5.3. Fibrin overlying the pupil.

Clinical Investigations

The objectives of performing investigations in uveitis patients are

- Confirmation of diagnosis — often the underlying aetiology is unknown but it is always important to rule out infective causes

- Aid in management — for monitoring of disease activity, efficacy of treatment and associated side effect(s)

Baseline investigations are required in patients who have bilateral uveitis on presentation or recurrent disease. Special investigations are ordered on a case-by-case basis.

Table 5.6. Clinical Investigations

	Investigation	Possible Aetiology(ies)
Baseline	• Full blood count (FBC) • Erythrocyte sedimentation rate (ESR) • Syphilis serology • Mantoux, T-Spot.TB or TB quantiferon • Chest X-ray • Urinalysis	
Special (systemic)	• ANA, anti ds-DNA • Serum ACE, CT Thorax • ANCA • HLA-B27 • Toxoplasma serology	• Vasculitis work-up • Sarcoidosis • Granulomatosis with polyangiitis • HLA-B27 associated disease • Toxoplasmosis
Special (ocular)	• FFA and ICG • Endothelial cell count • Aqueous tap and PCR • Vitreous biopsy	• Posterior uveitis • Hypertensive uveitis

When there is a suspicion of possible infective aetiology, or any associated underlying connective tissue disease or oncological condition, such cases should be co-managed with the relevant specialists prior to initiating any treatment

Patients who require immunosuppression therapy may need to be co-managed with the rheumatologist

Management

Uveitis is a challenging condition to treat and the aim is to abolish the underlying inflammation which could result from various infectious and non-infectious aetiologies

The basic therapeutic principles are:

• To treat specific infectious causes such as ocular tuberculosis, syphilis, viral retinitis (e.g. acute retinal necrosis or CMV retinitis, toxoplasmosis, endophthalmitis);

• To treat non-infectious uveitis with corticosteroids (systemic or topical);

• To consider the use of immunomodulatory agents if the patient has suffered steroid-induced complications, when steroids are not tolerated or contraindicated, in the presence of frequent flare-ups on tapering steroids , or if the underlying uveitis are associated with an ocular or systemic condition for which immunomodulatory agents are clinically indicated (e.g. Behçet's disease, granulomatosis with polyangiitis).

Treatment Modalities

Steroids

These are available in various formulations

Topical steroids, e.g. prednisolone acetate 1%, are typically indicated for anterior chamber inflammation

Periocular or intravitreal steroids, e.g. triamcinolone (periocular or intravitreal), OZURDEX® (dexamethasone intravitreal implant), can be considered in cases of intermediate uveitis with significant inflammation and cystoid macular oedema. Systemic steroids are used either as an adjunct to treatment for specific aetiologies or as a primary treatment, for bilateral or severe intermediate or posterior uveitis

Cycloplegics

For example, atropine 1% or the less potent homatropine 1% eyedrop. This acts to stabilise the blood aqueous barrier and to break existing posterior synechiae. Adding a mydriatic such as phenylephrine 2.5% or 10% can act synergistically with a cycloplegic to break the posterior synechiae

Immunomodulatory Agents

For example, azathioprine, methotrexate, mycophenolate mofetil, tacrolimus, infliximab , adalimumab, have been used in uveitis. (Details of these agents are beyond the scope of this chapter)

Complications

Anterior Segment Complications

Iris

Posterior synechiae that is extensive could lead to seclusio pupillae (Fig. 5.4) and increase the risk of secondary angle closure from pupil block. Early administration of cycloplegics and mydriatics play a role in breaking existing posterior synechiae

Iris atrophy can be a diagnostic feature of herpetic uveitis. Sector iris atrophy is seen in zoster-related uveitis

The following pictures demonstrate the effects of cycloplegics and mydriatics in an uveitic eye with seclusio pupillae (Fig. 5.5)

Surgical iridectomy may sometimes be indicated in eyes which have failed to respond to pharmacological measures and where the intraocular pressures remain elevated in the presence of maximal tolerated medical treatment

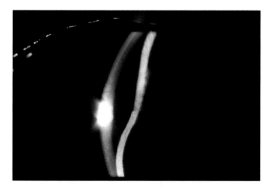

Fig. 5.4. Secondary angle closure with pupil block from seclusio pupillae.

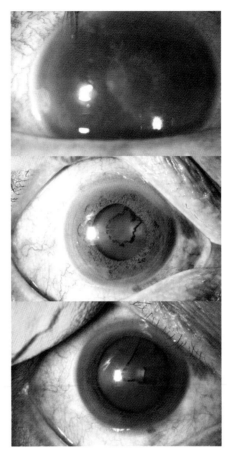

Fig. 5.5. (From top to bottom) the effects of cycloplegics and mydriatics in an uveitic eye with seclusio pupillae.

Intraocular pressure (IOP)

Low IOP may results from ciliary body shutdown in active or uncontrolled ocular inflammation

Factors that result in elevated IOP include peripheral anterior synechiae formation, which results in secondary angle closure or from various causes of secondary open angle mechanisms such as steroid therapy, trabeculitis or accumulation of inflammatory material and debris in the trabecular meshwork

Anterior chamber

Inflammatory ciliochoroidal effusion (e.g. in Vogt-Koyanagi-Harada disease) can give rise to shallow anterior chambers which usually improve with systemic steroids or immunotherapy

Lens

Cataract may develop due to a combination of factors which include inflammation (recurrent or chronic) or the long term use of steroids

Posterior segment complications

Macula

Anterior and posterior segment inflammation or chronic inflammation can lead to cystoid macular oedema, exudative macular detachment and choroidal neovascular membrane

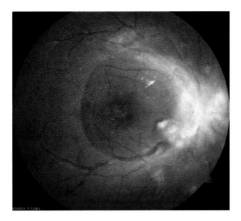

Fig. 5.6. Optic disc infiltrated with sarcoid granulomas.

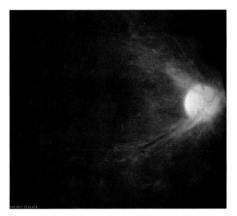

Fig. 5.7. Resolution of optic disc granulomas with treatment.

Optic nerve

Optic disc inflammation can occur isolated or concurrently with other signs of anterior and posterior uveitis. Sometimes isolated optic disc swelling may be observed in cases of posterior scleritis. Sarcoid granulomas can infiltrate the optic disc and give the appearance of a disc swelling (Fig. 5.6 and Fig. 5.7)

Retina

Retinitis and vasculitis can sometimes lead to occlusive vasculitis and consequently, vascular occlusion with its attendant problems such as neovascularisation

Exudative retinal detachment may also occur in some instances of uveitis

Take home messages
- A systematic approach to assessing a patient with uveitis is paramount and this includes a detailed history and thorough ocular examination.
- The initial assessment will then guide the clinician on the necessary investigations.
- Investigations will aid the management of a patient with uveitis.
- Certain uveitis cases may require co-management with internal physicians such as rheumatologists and infectious disease specialists.

5.3 Toxoplasmosis

Learning Objectives
• Understanding the clinical manifestation of congenital and acquired toxoplasmosis.
• Understanding the management of ocular toxoplasmosis.

• *Toxoplasma gondii* is an obligate intracellular parasite
• Transmission of the protozoa varies demographically — consumption of raw or undercooked meat in more developed countries versus drinking untreated water in under-developed countries
• Cats are the definitive hosts whereas humans and livestock are intermediate hosts
• The oocysts excreted in cat faeces become encysted (bradyzoite) or actively proliferating (tachyzoite) upon ingestion
• Congenital toxoplasmosis from vertical transmission is more severe if contracted early in the pregnancy

Clinical Presentation

Patients with toxoplasmosis can have either of the following presentation:
• Bilateral poor vision with strabismus — congenital toxoplasmosis typically causes bilateral retinochoroiditis affecting the macula resulting in poor vision and strabismus
• Acute onset blurring of vision with floaters — acquired toxoplasmosis is often asymptomatic and can affect both eyes in 40% of cases. It is imperative to maintain a low index of suspicion for immunocompromised status in bilateral, simultaneously active cases with large and / or multiple lesions

Table 5.7. Clinical Presentation of Ocular Toxoplasmosis

Ophthalmic	Systemic
Symptoms • Blurring of vision • Floaters **Signs** • Vitritis with retinitis (classic 'headlight in a fog' appearance) – retinitis is white and fluffy in appearance and may be adjacent to an previous toxoplasmosis scar (Figs. 5.8, 5.9), satellite lesions adjacent to the scar are also commonly seen • Others: scleritis, neuroretinitis, serous retinal detachment, punctate outer retinal toxoplasmosis (PORT) **Complications** • Cataract • Glaucoma • Choroidal neovascularisation	**Congenital** • Hydrocephalus • Cerebral calcification • Hepatosplenomegaly • Retinochoroiditis **Acquired** • Fever • Lymphadenopathy • NB: if immunocomprised there is risk of life-threatening disease e.g. encephalitis, intracerebral cysts, hepatitis, myocarditis

Patients with a history of ocular toxoplasmosis presenting with new onset blurring vision or floaters, whether in the affected or fellow eye, warrant an urgent ophthalmology referral

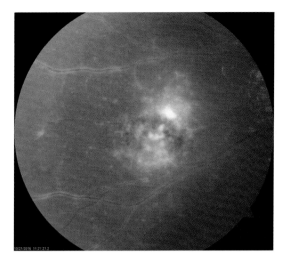

Fig. 5.8. Active retinochoroiditis with vasculitis adjacent to an old toxoplasmosis scar.

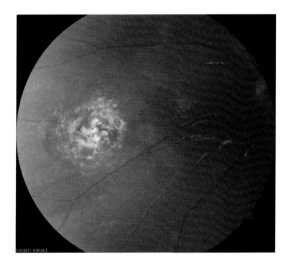

Fig. 5.9. Toxoplasmosis scar.

Clinical Investigation

Ocular toxoplasmosis is a clinical diagnosis. However, it is important to exclude other causes of retinitis, in which case PCR of intraocular fluid is useful. Toxoplasma serology is useful but should be interpreted with care, as anti-toxoplasma IgG are positive in many adults. The presence of IgM antibodies suggests acquired infection

Clinical Management

Indications for treatment:

- Lesion(s) involving the optic disc, macula or papillomacular bundle
- Lesion(s) threatening major vessels
- Lesion(s) larger than 1 disc diameter in size
- Marked vitritis
- Immunocompromised patients

Various treatment regimens are available:

- Prednisolone + sulphadiazine + pyrimethamine + folinic acid (this is the classic "triple therapy" with folinic acid supplementation)
- Prednisolone + sulphadiazine + pyrimethamine + clindamycin + folinic acid ("quadruple therapy")
- Prednisolone + co-trimoxazole
- Prednisolone + clindamycin
- Prednisolone + atovaquone
- Prednisolone + azithromycin

Systemic steroids are typically commenced at least 24 hours after initiation of anti-toxoplasmosis therapy. Patients are co-managed with the infectious disease specialist. In the case of pregnant patients, the obstetrician should be involved in the management as well

In immunocompetent patients, the disease is self-limiting, hence, treatment is only required for sight-threatening lesions. Recurrence is possible and patients should be informed

All patients require regular follow-up until resolution of the disease, which is seen as complete scarring with resolution of inflammation. Patients should be advised to seek medical attention should they develop blurring of vision or floaters upon discharge

Take home messages

- Ocular toxoplasmosis is a potentially sight-threatening condition, e.g. in immunocompromised patients, or lesions involving the macula.
- Ocular toxoplasmosis is a clinical diagnosis however investigations are occasionally required to rule out other causes.
- Acute ocular toxoplasmosis is often co-managed by ophthalmologists and infectious disease specialists.
- Special attention must be paid to pregnant patients with acute ocular toxoplasmosis.

5.4 Cytomegalovirus Retinitis

Learning Objectives
- Understanding the clinical presentation of CMV retinitis.
- Understanding the management of CMV retinitis.

Cytomegalovirus (CMV) is a double-stranded DNA virus belonging to the Herpesviridae family. CMV retinitis can be seen in immunocompromised patients with malignancy (e.g. lymphoma or leukaemia, post-transplant patients, and retroviral positive individuals.)

CMV retinitis occurs in up to 40% of AIDS cases, typically when the CD4 count falls under $50/mm^3$.

Clinical Presentation

Patients may be asymptomatic, particularly if the retinitis does not involve the macula. Screening is therefore important especially when the CD4 count is low

Severely immunocompromised patients are often unable to mount any immune response, hence, the absence of ocular inflammation. On the contrary, marked immune response can be seen in immune reconstitution uveitis (IRU) upon recovery of the immune system, typically seen after initiation of highly active antiretroviral therapy (HAART)

Table 5.8. Ocular Presentation of CMV Retinitis

Symptoms	• Blurring of vision • Visual field loss • Floaters

Signs	Anterior
	• Anterior chamber inflammation – mild or typically absent
	
	Posterior
	• Vitritis – mild or typically absent
	
	Retinitis – 3 variants have been described
	• Classic or fulminant retinitis
	  • Classic "tomato and cheese" appearance with retinal haemorrhage and yellowish, fluffy retinitis often seen in the posterior pole from the optic disc (Fig. 5.10) along the arcade in the distribution of the retinal nerve fibre layer
	• Granular or indolent form
	  • Typically found in the peripheral retina
	  • Minimal or no haemorrhage or retinal oedema or vasculitis
	  • Active retinitis along edge of the lesion
	• Perivascular form
	  • A variant of frosted branch angiitis – idiopathic retinal perivasculitis

Complications	• Retinal detachment (up to 30%) • Retinal atrophy • Optic nerve disease

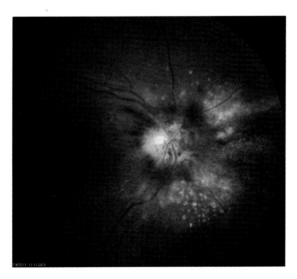

Fig. 5.10. CMV retinitis with optic disc involvement.

Clinical Investigations

CMV retinitis is a clinical diagnosis. Baseline blood investigations are performed for monitoring of treatment and side effects (e.g. agranulocytosis from ganciclovir)

Clinical Management

A multi-disciplinary approach is essential

Treatment

- HAART for HIV patients: to sustain CD4 count above 50mm^3
- Anti-CMV treatment: this involves "induction" and "maintenance" regime. Combination therapy may be required depending on disease severity.
  - Systemic: valganciclovir, ganciclovir, foscarnet, cidofovir
  - Intravitreal: ganciclovir, foscarnet
  - Intravitreal implant: ganciclovir

Patients should be monitored for immune recovery uveitis and retinal detachment.

> **Take home messages**
> - CMV infection can be congenital or acquired.
> - A high index of suspicion must be maintained in patients with AIDS having CD4 count <50/mm^3 or other immunocompromised status, e.g. following bone marrow or organ transplant.
> - Immunocompromised patients may be completely asymptomatic.
> - Referral to ophthalmology is paramount when there is a CD4 count <50/mm^3 or when there is any clinical suspicion.

5.5 Endogenous Endophthalmitis

> **Learning Objectives**
> - Understanding the clinical presentation of endophthalmitis.
> - Understanding the management of endophthalmitis.

Endogenous endophthalmitis is an intraocular infection arising from haematogenous dissemination of bacterial or fungal organisms from a remote primary source, typically from liver abscesses or urinary tract infections. Although endogenous endophthalmitis is uncommon, it is a potentially blinding condition and should always be considered as a differential for acute, painful, red eye with blurring of vision.

Who is at Risk?

- Immunocompromised patients
- Predisposing conditions
  - Diabetes mellitus
  - Systemic malignancy
  - Sickle cell anaemia
  - AIDS
  - Extensive gastrointestinal surgery
- Potential sources of infection
  - Pneumonia
  - Urinary tract infection
  - Bacterial meningitis
  - Liver abscess

Table 5.9. Common Pathogens Causing Endogenous Endophthalmitis

Bacterial	Fungal
Gram positive organisms • *Streptococcus species* (endocarditis) • *Staphylococcus* aureus (cutaneous infection) • Bacillus species (IVDU)	• *Candida albicans, Candida glabrata* • *Aspergillus fumigatus* • *Cryptococcus neoformans* • *Coccidioides immitis*
Gram negative organisms • *Neisseria meningitides* • *Haemophilus influenza* • Enteric organisms (e.g. *Klebsiella species, Escherichia coli*)	

Clinical Presentation

Bacterial endophthalmitis tends to present acutely with pain whereas fungal endophthalmitis tends to develop slowly and may be painless

Table 5.10. Ocular Presentation of Endogenous Endophthalmitis

Symptoms	• Pain • Photophobia • Blurring of vision
Signs	• Severely reduced vision • Periorbital and eyelid oedema • Anterior chamber fibrin, hypoypon • Vitritis • Choroiditis (Fig. 5.11), retinitis ± necrosis
Complications	• Retinal detachment • Vitreous haemorrhage, suprachoroidal haemorrhage • Hypotony • Pthisis bulbi

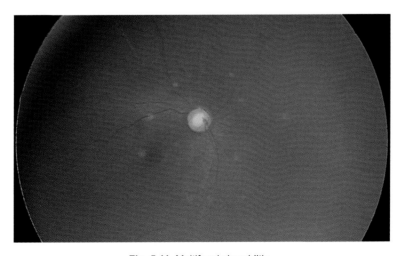

Fig. 5.11. Multifocal choroiditis.

Management

Confirmation of diagnosis

• Blood culture

• Ocular culture: vitreous tap

Endogenous endopthalmitis is sight threatening and rapid commencement of empirical anti-microbial treatment is crucial. If fungal endophthalmitis is suspected, concurrent anti-bacterial and anti-fungal treatment is initiated. Depending on the severity, combination of systemic and intravitreal treatment may be required

Prognosis is dependent on the organism and the immune status of the patient

Take home messages

• Endogenous endophthalmitis is a serious, potentially blinding condition.

• It is commonly caused by haematogenous dissemination of bacterial or fungal organisms.

• The most common bacterial organism in the South East Asia region is Klebsiella spp.

• Patients with systemic infections secondary to the organisms listed especially Klebsiella spp. must be referred to an ophthalmologist for screening.

5.6 Systemic Diseases Associated Uveitis

Learning Objectives

Identify the systemic diseases associated with uveitis and its management.

Juvenile Idiopathic Arthritis (JIA)

Juvenile idiopathic arthritis (JIA)-associated uveitis is a challenging condition whereby both inflammation and treatment might result in problems that present themselves to the Ophthalmologist. Medical and surgical treatment options might have to be considered in the management of these problems. A multidisciplinary approach is often required in the management of JIA (International League of Associations for Rheumatology (ILAR) nomenclature), also known as juvenile rheumatoid arthritis.

American College of Rheumatology Criteria for Juvenile Rheumatoid Arthritis

JRA can be diagnosed if age at onset is under 16 years; there is arthritis in 1 or more joints; disease duration is 6 weeks or greater; and other forms of juvenile arthritis (e.g. psoriatic and inflammatory bowel disease-associated arthritis) excluded.

Disease type is defined by the type of disease present in the first 6 months.

• Systemic-onset JRA: daily (quotidian) fever spiking to more than 39°C (102.2°F) for 2 weeks or greater in association with arthritis of 1 or more joints.

• Pauciarticular JRA: arthritis in 4 or fewer joints in the first 6 months of disease.

• Polyarticular JRA: arthritis in 5 or more joints in the first 6 months of disease.

Risk Factors for Developing Uveitis

JIA-associated uveitis is usually described as chronic, bilateral, non-granulomatous anterior uveitis, with an insidious onset. As this is usually asymptomatic, screening for JIA-associated uveitis in at-risk patients is important. Majority of cases are diagnosed within 4 years from the onset of arthritis

Risk factors for the development of uveitis
- Oligoarticular arthritis
- Young age at the onset of the disease
- Antinuclear antibodies (ANA) seropositivity
- Rheumatoid factor (RF) seronegativity
- Female gender

Complications of JIA-associated Uveitis

- Band-shaped Keratopathy
- Cataract
- Glaucoma
- Hypotony
- Epiretinal membrane
- Macular oedema

Treatment Options

- Topical glucocorticoids and cycloplegics
- Immunosuppressants (e.g. methotrexate)
- Biological therapy

HLA-B27-associated Acute Anterior Uveitis

HLA-B27-associated acute anterior uveitis is relatively common.

It has been estimated that up to 20% of people carrying the HLA-B27 antigen have at least one of the several following associated conditions, which include:
- Ankylosing spondylitis
- Reactive arthritis (including Reiter's syndrome)
- Psoriatic arthritis
- Undifferentiated spondyloarthropathies
- Enteropathic arthropathy
- Inflammatory bowel disease

It is, therefore, important to take a detailed history and to conduct a directed systemic examination of these patients

Classically, HLA-B27 associated acute anterior uveitis presents as a sudden onset, acute anterior uveitis in a young patient, typically male. It starts in one eye but is usually asymmetrically bilateral. The inflammation may be associated with a fibrinous reaction, hypopyon and the formation of posterior synechiae

These patients typically respond readily to topical corticosteroid therapy

Take home messages

• Juvenile idiopathic arthritis is associated with chronic uveitis and its complications in younger patients.

• HLA-B27 associated uveitis should be co-managed with a rheumatologist so that the systemic conditions can be addressed.

5.7 Scleritis and Episcleritis

Learning Objectives

Identify and differentiate scleritis from episcleritis.

Differentiation between the two entities is important as the manifestations, prognosis and complications differ.

Episcleritis refers to inflammation confined to the superficial episcleral tissue whereas scleritis refers to the inflammation of the sclera which might involve other ocular structures such as the adjacent cornea.

Episcleritis is non-vision threatening, usually idiopathic and can be self-limiting.

Aetiologies

The most common systemic associations of scleritis include rheumatoid arthritis, granulomatosis with polyangiitis, relapsing polycondritis and polyarteritis nodosa.

Infectious scleritis can be bacterial, viral, fungal or parasitic

Surgically induced necrotising scleritis (SINS) can occur following a variety of procedures

Investigations

In scleritis (Figs. 5.12, 5.13), these have to be tailored to exclude infectious causes and systemic associations

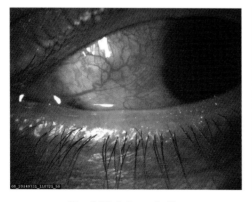

Fig. 5.12. Active scleritis.

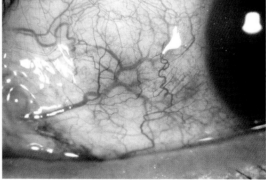

Fig. 5.13. Resolved scleritis with area of scleral thinning.

Treatment

Non-steroidal anti-inflammatory agents

Non-selective cox inhibitors such as indomethacin or ibuprofen can first be considered in the absence of any contraindications

Gastrointestinal side effects and renal toxicity from the use of non-steroidal anti-inflammatory agents are some important considerations

Corticosteroids

Steroids are commenced for those who do not respond to non-steroidal anti-inflammatory agents, posterior or necrotising disease. Systemic corticosteroids may be given orally or intravenously

Steroid-sparing agents

In the presence of contraindications or intolerance to steroids or patients who relapse at doses of prednisolone >7.5mg–10mg per day, adjunctive immunosuppressive therapy should be considered. Options include methotrexate and azathioprine

Take home messages

Scleritis is associated with more ocular morbidity and should be investigated and managed with anti-inflammatory drugs.

References

1. Abu Samra K et al. (2016) Current treatment modalities of JIA-associated uveitis and its complications: Literature review. *Ocul Immunol Inflamm* **24**(4):431–9.

2. Alistair K O Denniston, P I Murray. (2014) *Oxford Handbook of Ophthalmology. 3rd ed.* NY: Oxford University Press, pp.410–413.

3. Brewer EJ Jr, Bass J, Baum J, *et al.* (1977) Current proposed revision of JRA criteria. JRA criteria subcommittee of the diagnostic and therapeutic criteria committee of the American rheumatism section of the arthritis foundation. *Arthritis Rheum* **20**(2 Suppl):195–199.

4. British Society for Paediatric and Adolescent Rheumatology, Royal College of Ophthalmology.(2006) Guidelines for Screening for Uveitis in Juvenile Idiopathic Arthritis.

5. Chang JH *et al.* (2005) Acute anterior uveitis and HLA-B27. *Surv Ophthalmol* **50**(4):364–88.

6. Deschenes J *et al.* (2008) International Uveitis Study Group. International Uveitis Study Group (IUSG): clinical classification of uveitis. *Ocul Immunol Inflamm* **16**:1–2.

7. Intraocular Inflammation and Uveitis, Section 9. Basic and Clinical Science Course, AAO, 2016.

8. Jabs DA *et al.* (2005) Standardisation of Uveitis Nomenclature (SUN) for reporting clinical data. *Am J Ophthalmol* **140**:509–16.

9. N Okhravi, *et al.* (2005) Scleritis. *Surv Ophthalmol* **50** :351–363.

10. Smith JR. (2002) HLA-B27--associated uveitis. *Ophthalmol Clin North Am* **15**(3):297—307.

11. Yang P, *et al.* (2011) Vogt-Koyanagi-Harada disease presenting as acute angle closure glaucoma at onset. *Clin Exp Ophthalmol* **39**(7):639—47

Chapter 6

VITREORETINAL DISORDERS

6.1 Inherited Retinal Disorders

Learning Objectives
• Introduction to retinitis pigmentosa.
• Appreciate fundus changes in retinitis pigmentosa.
• Understand syndromes associated with retinitis pigmentosa.

Retinitis Pigmentosa

• Retinitis pigmentosa (RP) refers to a group of inherited disorders that affect the photoreceptor/retinal pigment epithelium (RPE) layers

• Classically, patients complain of poor night vision. As the disease progresses, they may lose vision in the affected eye

• RP may present in many variants. One or both eyes can be affected and the severity of the fundus changes may vary between different variants

• In addition, the mode of inheritance also may differ with different age of onset

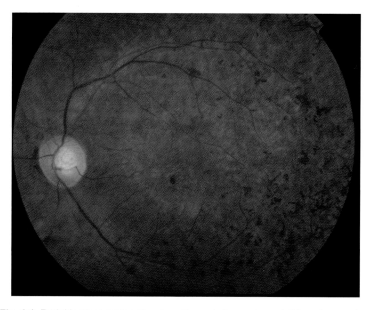

Fig. 6.1. Retinitis pigmentosa showing attenuated vessels and diffuse bony spicules.

115

"Typical" findings in retinitis pigmentosa (Fig. 6.1)
- Pigmentary retinal changes (bony spicules)
  - Can be generalised (affecting entire retina) or segmental (affect only a portion of the retina)
- Attenuated arteries
- Waxy pallor of optic nerve

Some forms of RP are associated with disorders in other parts of the body

- Usher's syndrome: RP and deafness
- Lawrence-Moon-Bardet-Biedl syndrome: RP and polydactyly

Other ocular findings in RP may include:

- Cataracts
- Cystoid macular oedema

At the time of printing, RP is generally managed conservatively with efforts focussed on maximising patients' vision with low vision aids and community support (e.g. Singapore Association of the Visually Handicapped). Research is ongoing and therapeutic options such as gene therapy and retinal implants are being studied

Take home messages

Retinitis pigmentosa is a progressive retinal disorder associated with contricted visual fields and nyctalopia.

6.2 Diabetic Retinopathy

Learning Objectives
- Classification of diabetic retinopathy.
- Understand mechanisms of vision loss due to diabetic retinopathy.
- Principles of management of diabetic retinopathy.

Concept of Ischaemic Drive

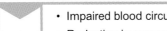
- Impaired blood circulation in eye from diabetes, retinal vein occlusion
- Reduction in oxygen supply to retina

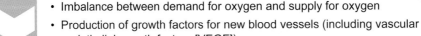
- Imbalance between demand for oxygen and supply for oxygen
- Production of growth factors for new blood vessels (including vascular endothelial growth factors [VEGF])

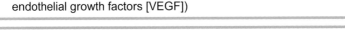
- New vessels grow in retina and anterior chamber
- Vitreous haemorrhage or neovascular glaucoma

Diabetic Retinopathy

Diabetic patients can develop macro and microvascular complications of diabetes mellitus throughout the body. Within the eye, diabetic changes can be classified based on:

- Severity of background retinopathy
- Presence or absence of diabetic macular disease

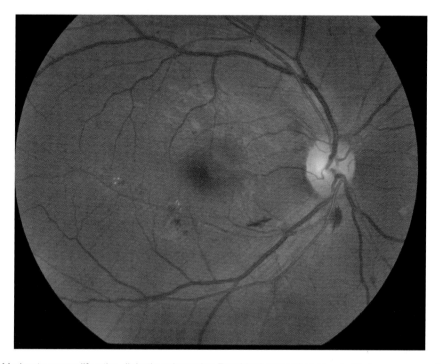

Fig. 6.2. Moderate nonproliferative diabetic retinopathy: Few blot haemorrhages noted but no new vessels seen.

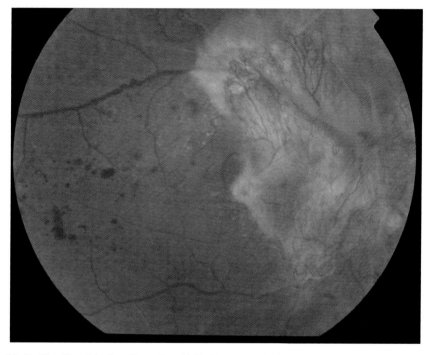

Fig. 6.3. Proliferative diabetic retinopathy with florid neovascularisation and fibrosis at the optic disc.

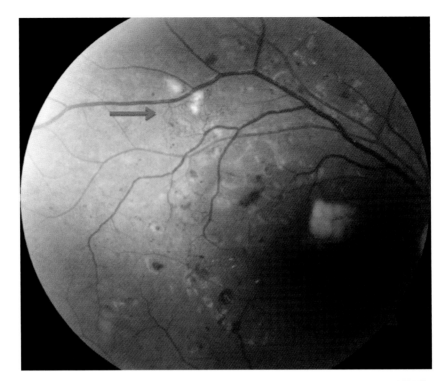

Fig. 6.4. Early new vessels seen.

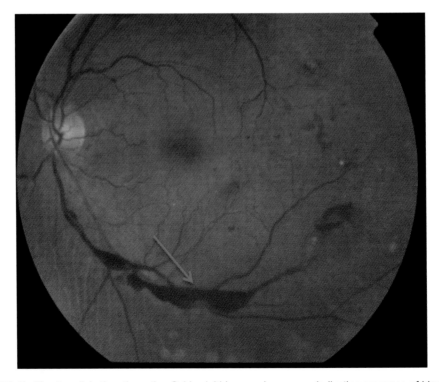

Fig. 6.5. Proliferative diabetic retinopathy: Subhyaloid haemorrhage seen indicating presence of bleeding from new vessels.

Background retinopathy
(ETDRS classification; Early Treatment of Diabetic Retinopathy Study)

Non proliferative diabetic retinopathy (NPDR)

- Mild NPDR
  - At least 1 microaneurysm, but not enough to qualify as moderate NPDR
- Moderate NPDR (Fig. 6.2)
  - Extensive intraretinal haemorrhages and/or microaneurysms, cotton wool spots, venous beading but not enough to qualify as severe NPDR
- Severe NPDR
  - Defined as "4-2-1" rule as any one of the following
    - i. Intraretinal haemorrhages and/or microaneurysms in all 4 quadrants
    - ii. Venous beading in at least 2 quadrants
    - iii. IRMA (Intraretinal microvascular abnormalities) in at least 1 quadrant

Proliferative diabetic retinopathy (PDR)

- Presence of new vessels on the disc (NVD) (Fig. 6.3)
- Presence of new vessels elsewhere (NVE) (Figs. 6.4, 6.5)

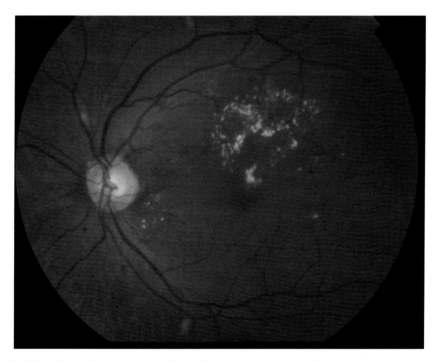

Fig. 6.6. Clinically significant macular oedema: Microaneurysms seen with surrounding hard exudates.

Clinically Significant Macular Oedema (CSME) (Fig. 6.6)

One of the following:

- Thickening within 500 µm of the fovea.
- Hard exudates within 500 µm of the fovea with associated retinal thickening.
- Area of retinal thickening of 1 disc area in size, any part of which is within 1 disc diameter of the fovea.

In many countries, diabetic eye screening is widely available via the use of the DRP (Diabetic Retinal Photography) programme. Fundus photos are taken and presence or absence of diabetic retinopathy is graded

Diagnosis and Classification

When examining the fundus, the severity of background diabetic retinopathy must be graded (either mild/mod/severe NPDR or PDR) as well as the presence or absence of macular disease (CSME)

Diabetic retinal disease can cause blurring of vision via a few mechanisms:

- Bleeding from new vessels resulting in:
  - Vitreous haemorrhage
  - Tractional retinal detachment
- Macular oedema from CSME
- Neovascular glaucoma

Treatment

Systemic treatment involves the management of the diabetic sugar levels. Tight control of blood sugar slows the progression of diabetic retinopathy. However, an important point to note is that rapid normalisation of the HbA1c after a period of prolonged poor diabetic control may paradoxically cause worsening of the macula oedema (Diabetes Control and Complications Trial)

With regards to the ocular management, treatment options depend on the severity of the background retinopathy as well as the presence/absence of CSME

Background retinopathy treatment
(ETDRS classification; Early Treatment of Diabetic Retinopathy Study)

Non proliferative diabetic retinopathy (NPDR)

Mild and moderate diabetic retinopathy is usually managed conservatively aside from encouraging good control of blood sugar levels.

Severe NPDR can also be observed. However, most doctors would initiate treatment via pan retinal photocoagulation (PRP; Fig. 6.7) by this stage to prevent visual loss.

Proliferative diabetic retinopathy (PDR)

PDR is managed with PRP

- PRP involves the application of laser burns in the retinal periphery to reduce the oxygen demand of the retina, therefore reducing the imbalance between poor oxygen supply from diseased retinal vessels and the high demand from the photoreceptors in the retina.

Tractional retinal detachment (TRD)

- TRD develops when new vessels that grow in PDR start to contract and pull on the retina. If the macula is involved, the tractional bands may cause vision to drop.

- Once the macula is involved by the TRD, surgery is usually indicated.

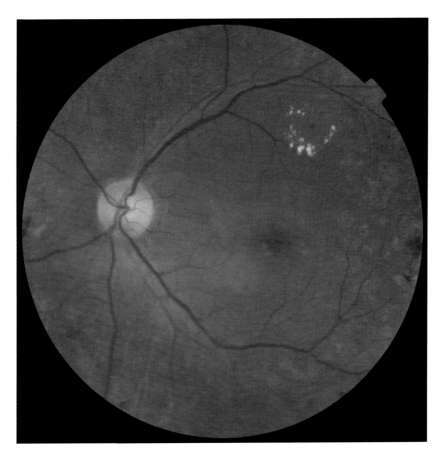

Fig. 6.7. Pan retinal photocoagulation laser scars are seen in the peripheral.

Clinically Significant Macular Oedema (CSME) treatment options

- Focal/Grid laser to leaking microaneurysms in the macula
  - Decreases risk of vision loss from macula oedema by 50% (ETDRS study)
- Intravitreal anti-vascular endothelial growth factor (Anti-VEGF)
  - Intravitreal injections of anti-VEGF has been shown in multiple studies to reduce the macula oedema and improve visual acuity in patients with diabetic macula oedema
  - At the time of publishing, 3 agents are available (Bevacizumab, Ranibizumab and Aflibercept). The application of bevacizumab for diabetic macular oedema is an off-label use but being significantly cheaper than the other 2 drugs, it is widely used

Take home messages

- Diabetic retinopathy can be classified into non-proliferative and proliferative stages.
- Treatment of diabetic retinopathy depends on the severity of disease based on ETDRS classification.
- The treatment of diabetic retinopathy and macular oedema should include both systemic and ocular approaches.

6.3 Retinal Vein Occlusions

Learning Objectives

- Branch retinal vein occlusions (BRVO) vs Central retinal vein occlusions (CRVO).
- Understand mechanisms of vision loss in retinal vein occlusions.
- Role of systemic illness in retinal vein occlusions.
- Principles of management of retinal vein occlusions.

The retinal veins allow blood to be drained from the retina and can be occluded at 2 sites:
- At or posterior to the lamina cribrosa (where the central retinal vein leaves the eyeball)
- At an arteriovenous crossing on the retina (where the vein shares a common adventitial sheath with a retinal artery)

Occlusion at the level of the lamina cribrosa obstructs the central retinal vein and results in a central retinal vein occlusion (CRVO; Fig. 6.8) whereas an obstruction at an arteriovenous crossing results in only a branch of the retinal veins being occluded (BRVO; Fig. 6.9)

Venous occlusion results in backflow of blood leading to the fundoscopic findings of multiple blot and flame shaped haemorrhages. Yellowish cotton wool spots, representing small infarcts of the nerve fibre layer, are also seen

Fundoscopic findings in a retinal vein occlusion

Acute presentation

- Scattered flame and blot hemorrhages in a segmental fashion (BRVO) or diffusely through the eye (CRVO)
- Cotton wool spots
- Dilated tortuous retinal veins
- Disc swelling

Chronic findings

- Sclerosed vein
- Opticiliary shunt
- Segmental / diffuse disc pallor
- Neovascularisation of the iris

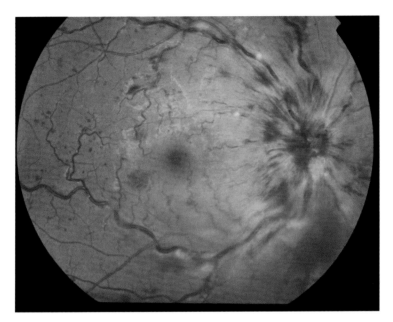

Fig. 6.8. Central retinal vein occlusion (disc swelling, dilated tortuous veins, scattered flame and blot haemorrhages, cotton wool spots).

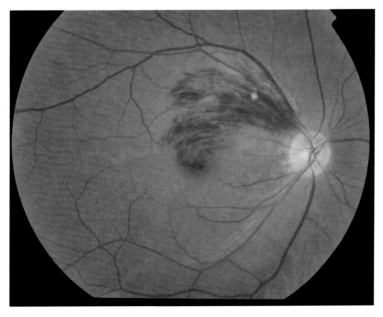

Fig. 6.9. Branch retinal vein occlusion (due to thickened atherosclerotic artery compressing on vein in the common shared adventitial sheath).

Vision Loss in Retinal Vein Occlusions

Vision loss can occur in a few ways

- Macula involvement
  - Macular oedema
  - Macular ischaemia
- Neovascular glaucoma (usually due to an ischaemic central retinal venous occlusion which leads to new vessel growth in the anterior segment which in turn leads to raised intraocular pressure)
- Vitreous haemorrhage from new vessels on the disc (NVD) or elsewhere (NVE)

Role of Systemic Diseases in Retinal Venous Occlusions

The roles of systemic diseases differ slightly in BRVO versus a CRVO.

In a BRVO, venous occlusion usually occurs at an arteriovenous crossing. Atherosclerosis leads to thickening of the arterial wall. This, in turn, causes compression of the vein at the site of crossing (Fig. 6.10) and induces the BRVO.

The main risk factors for a BRVO are

- Increasing age
- Systemic arterial hypertension
- History of smoking
- History of glaucoma

In CRVO, the main risk factors are slightly different

- Systemic hypertension
- Open angle glaucoma
- Diabetes mellitus
- Hyperlipidemia

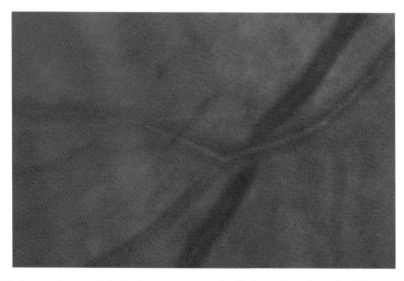

Fig. 6.10. This image shows a typical arteriovenous crossing in the retina where the thinner arterial vessel crosses a larger, dilated retinal vein.

Retinal vein occlusion treatment

Management strategies can be broadly divided into

- Identifying and treating systemic risk factors
- Identifying and treating ocular complications

Ocular complications

Macular oedema

- The mainstay of treatment is the use of intravitreal anti-VEGF agents or intravitreal steroids
- In BRVOs, grid laser may be attempted. Grid laser is not useful in CRVO associated macular oedema

Macular ischaemia

- Macular ischaemia is usually untreatable and has a grim prognosis for the patient's vision
- Low vision aids may be used for severe visual loss

Neovascular glaucoma

- A high threshold of suspicion must be maintained to identify and treat neovascular glaucoma early
- The mainstay in management is to reduce the ischaemic drive by performing laser photocoagulation to the ischaemic retina in the periphery
- Intravitreal anti-VEGF agents can also be used to reduce the high anti-VEGF levels and hopefully regress the new vessels that have appeared
- Anti-glaucoma eye drops are also started to reduce the intraocular pressure

Take home messages

- Vision loss from retinal vein occlusion can occur from macula involvement, neovascular glaucoma and vitreous haemorrhage.
- For macular oedema due to retinal vein occlusion, the mainstay of treatment is the use of intravitreal anti-VEGF agents or intravitreal steroids.

6.4 Retinal Artery Occlusions

Learning Objectives

- Branch retinal artery occlusions vs Central retinal artery occlusions.
- Understand mechanisms of vision loss in retinal artery occlusions.
- Role of systemic illness in retinal artery occlusions.
- Principles of management of retinal artery occlusions.

The central retinal artery supplies blood to the inner layers of the retina and can cause sudden visual loss if occluded (CRAO: Central retinal artery occlusion; Fig. 6.11). Some patients (approximately 20%) are fortunate enough to have a cilioretinal artery which arises from the choroidal circulation. If a patient with a CRAO has a concomitant cilioretinal artery, blood flow to the macula may be preserved and therefore, central vision may survive.

Retinal artery occlusion can occur along its branches as well (BRAO: Branch retinal artery occlusion; Fig. 6.12) causing a sudden onset partial visual loss in the affected segment

Fundoscopic findings in a retinal artery occlusion

Acute presentation
- Retinal whitening
- Cherry red spot
- The offending emboli may be seen (Cholesterol aka Hollenhorst plaques, platelet fibrin, calcific emboli)

Chronic findings
- Disc pallor

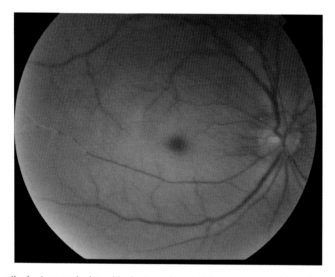

Fig. 6.11. Central retinal artery occlusion with cherry red spot, diffuse oedema. This patient underwent an anterior chamber paracentesis and had the retinal artery emboli dislodged to the inferiotemporal branch of the retinal artery.

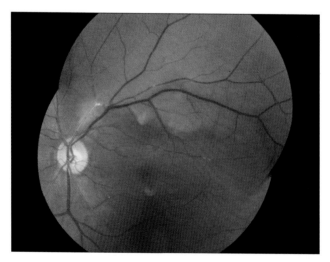

Fig. 6.12. Branch retinal artery occlusion with emboli seen in the retinal artery and retinal oedema in the area supplied by the blocked artery.

Role of Systemic Diseases in Retinal Artery Occlusions

Three main types of emboli have been described:

- Cholesterol emboli (Hollenhorst plaques) from the carotid arteries
- Platelet-fibrin emboli from atherosclerotic vessels
- Calcific emboli from abnormal cardiac valves

Generally, the underlying aetiology for a retinal artery occlusion varies depending on the patient's age. Carotid artery atherosclerosis is the most common aetiology in older patients

In younger patients, the development of a retinal artery occlusion prompts a systemic evaluation for an underlying cause

Potential causes may include:

i. Collagen vascular diseases (Giant cell arteritis, systemic lupus erythematosus)

ii. Prothrombotic conditions (Protein C/S deficiency, antithrombin III deficiency, oral contraceptives, pregnancy, cancer, hematological malignancies)

iii. Cardiac emboli

Retinal artery occlusion treatment

Management strategies can be broadly divided into:

- Identifying and treating systemic risk factors
- Acute management to dislodge the emboli to improve retinal circulation

Acute ocular intervention (aimed at dislodging clot)

- Digital ocular massage
- Carbogen inhalation
- Anterior chamber paracentesis
- Intravenous carbonic anhydrase inhibitor and other topical anti-glaucoma medications

Take home messages

- Retinal artery occlusion is an ocular emergency and should be identified promptly.
- The condition is associated with poor prognosis.

6.5 Hypertensive Retinopathy

Learning Objectives

Classification of hypertensive retinopathy.

Hypertension has effects on the precapillary arterioles in the eye

Early stages of hypertensive changes may include:

- Diffuse/focal retinal arteriolar narrowing
- Arteriolar wall opacification (Silver/Copper wiring)
- Compression of the venules at the arteriovenous junction (AV nicking/nipping)

Traditionally, the Keith-Wagener-Barker classification has been used to characterise these changes

Keith-Wagener-Barker classification

Grade 1

Mild generalised arteriolar narrowing/sclerosis

Grade 2

Generalised/focal arteriolar narrowing, silver/copper wiring, AV nicking/nipping (Fig. 6.10)

Grade 3

Haemorrhages (dot/blot/flame), microaneurysms, cotton wool spots, hard exudates (Fig. 6.13)

Grade 4 (Malignant hypertension)

Moderate changes + Disc swelling

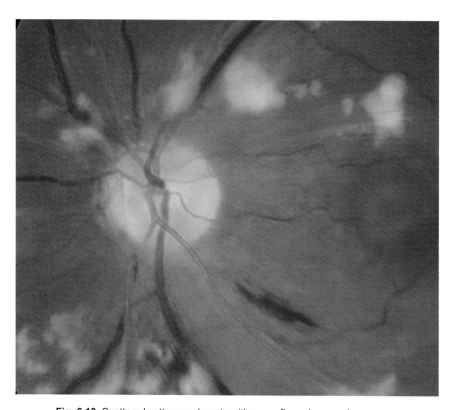

Fig. 6.13. Scattered cotton wool spots with some flame haemorrhages seen.

Take home messages

Hypertensive retinopathy can be classified based on the Keith-Wagener-Baker classification.

6.6 Age-related Macular Degeneration

Learning Objectives
- Difference between dry and wet age related macular degeneration (AMD).
- Understand mechanisms of vision loss in AMD.
- Role of smoking in AMD.
- Principles of management of AMD.

Age related macular degeneration (AMD) is a leading cause of central visual loss in persons above the age of 50. The hallmark finding in eyes with AMD is the presence of drusen in the macula.

Other findings may include:

  i. Retinal pigment layer abnormalities (geographic atrophy)

  ii. Haemorrhage

  iii. Disciform scarring

Classically, AMD has been divided into "dry" and "wet" forms. The dry form is characterised by presence of drusen in the macula which are initially visually asymptomatic (Fig. 6.14). Later on, atrophic macular scarring may develop (geographic atrophy; Fig. 6.15). The progression to macular scarring is a chronic process and does not involve the formation of any abnormal choroidal neovascular membrane (CNVM)

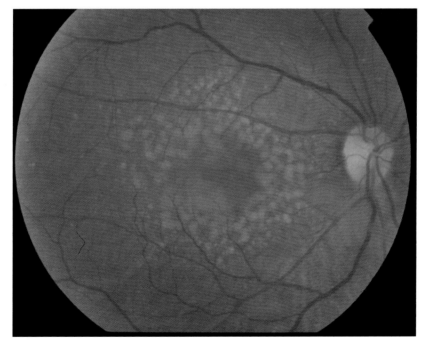

Fig. 6.14. Dry AMD with drusen seen around macula.

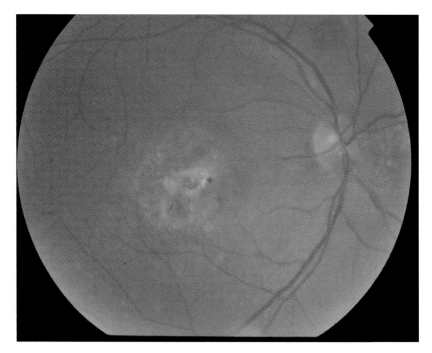

Fig. 6.15. Dry AMD with macula scar seen (also known as geographic atrophy).

In wet AMD, a CNVM forms at the macula. Histopathologically, these CNVM may lie above or below the retinal pigment epithelium (RPE). The actual formation of the CNVM is visually asymptomatic. However, these CNVM typically bleed (Fig. 6.16); causing a sudden drop in vision. Visual loss may manifest as mild metamorphopsia (due to the distortion in the photoreceptor layer from the oedema and bleeding) or may be more severe with sudden loss of central vision (due to a thick layer of blood over the photoreceptors)

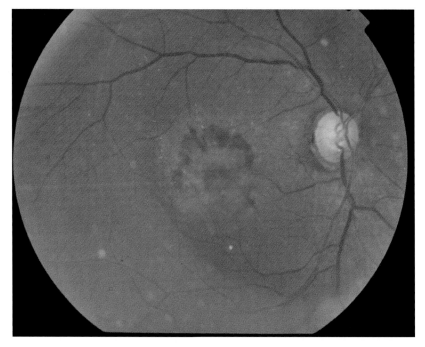

Fig. 6.16. Wet AMD: Haemorrhage noted in macula with surrounding drusen.

With regards to prevention, the main modifiable risk factor is smoking. Smoking cessation is currently an important aspect of management of any form of AMD

In addition, vitamin supplementation in the form of the AREDS (age-related eye disease) vitamins have been shown to help in reducing the progression to advanced AMD in some patients. At 10 years, 44% of placebo patients compared to 34% of the patients receiving the AREDS supplementation developed advanced AMD (a 27% risk reduction)

However, this benefit was noted in only two groups of patients:

    i. Individuals with intermediate AMD (extensive intermediate or at least 1 large drusen, or nonsubfoveal geographic atrophy)

    ii. Individuals with advanced unilateral AMD (vision loss due to AMD in one eye)

Regular surveillance with an Amsler grid (Fig. 6.17) is important. Patients are instructed to close one eye and focus on the central dot in the Amsler grid and report to their doctor if they have a sudden distortion/disappearance of the lines on the Amsler grid

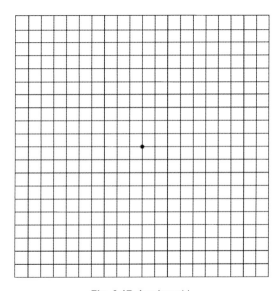

Fig. 6.17. Amsler grid.

Once the neovascular complications of AMD develop with hemorrhage and oedema in the macula seen, the mainstay of treatment then shifts to the use of intravitreal injections of anti-vascular endothelial growth factors (anti-VEGF). There are various anti-VEGFs available and common examples include:

- Bevacizumab (Avastin)
- Ranibizumab (Lucentis)
- Aflibercept (Eylea)

These injections are generally safe but carry a small risk of endophthalmitis with each injection. In addition, there are some concerns regarding the use of anti-VEGF agents in patients with a recent history of stroke or heart attacks

In some cases, laser therapy using Photodynamic Therapy (PDT) may be done. This involves the injection of a photosensitive drug into a peripheral vein which is then activated by a laser with a specific wavelength in the retina circulation. The activated drug then creates free radicals which then cause local damage in the abnormal retinal vasculature where it is activated

Take home messages

- Age-related macular degeneration can be classified into "dry" and "wet" forms.
- The underlying pathophysiology is related to choroidal neovascularisation.
- The mainstay of treatment is the use of intravitreal injections of anti-vascular endothelial growth factors (anti-VEGF) for exudative disease.

6.7 Retinal Tears/Retinal Detachments

Learning Objectives

- Understanding symptoms of a retinal tear.
- Development of a retinal detachment after a retinal tear.
- Role of early detection and prophylactic treatment of retinal tears.

Retinal tears are full thickness tears of the neurosensory retina. Typically, these tears are believed to occur due to traction from the vitreous body pulling on the retina causing a tear. This tractional force is especially strong once a posterior vitreous detachment develops.

To understand a posterior vitreous detachment, one must first understand that the vitreous body has an outer cortex, which, in the posterior part, is known as the posterior vitreous cortex. This posterior vitreous cortex is adherent to the surface of the retina. With age, the gel in the vitreous body starts to degenerate and liquefy, causing a drop in volume of the vitreous body. This leads to a contraction in the vitreous body and a subsequent detachment of its posterior cortex off the surface of the retina. This process is known as a posterior vitreous detachment (PVD).

When a PVD develops, patients typically experience floaters or photopsia. Once these symptoms develop, they should undergo a dilated fundus exam to ensure that retinal tears did not develop as the vitreous detachment occurred.

Left untreated, a tear provides an entry point for liquefied vitreous to enter the potential space between the neurosensory retina and the retinal pigment epithelium. As the liquefied vitreous enters this potential space, a neurosensory detachment occurs (retinal detachment) which can lead to visual field defects and eventually loss of central vision when the macula is involved.

Once a retinal detachment occurs, surgery is typically required. This may include options such as a pneumatic retinopexy, vitrectomy or scleral buckle procedure.

However, if the patient is diagnosed early before the retinal tear has converted to a retinal detachment (Fig. 6.18), prophylactic laser retinopexy (Fig. 6.19) can be done to surround the retinal tear with laser burns to seal the neurosensory retina to the retinal pigment epithelium. These lasers scars then prevent further movement of the liquefied vitreous gel thru the tear therefore preventing a retinal detachment.

There is no symptom that can distinguish which patient has a retinal tear or not. Only a dilated fundus exam is adequate in picking up a retinal tear.

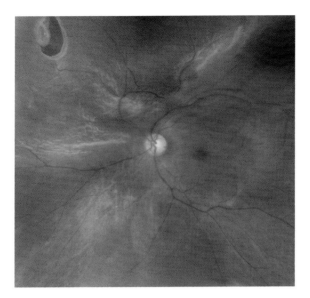

Fig. 6.18. Retinal detachment with horse shoe retinal tear seen superonasally.

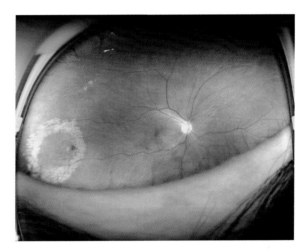

Fig. 6.19. Inferiotemporal retinal tear surrounded by fresh laser retinopexy burns.

Take home messages

Retinal detachment is an emergency and surgical intervention is associated with high rates of success.

References

1. American Academy of Ophthalmology (Basic and Clinical Sciences Course)
2. Hayrey SS, Zimmerman MB. (2014) Branch retinal vein occlusion: Natural history of visual outcome. *JAMA Ophthalmol* **132**(1)13–22.
3. *Kanski's Clinical Ophthalmology.*
4. The Diabetic Retinopathy Study Research Group. (1976) Preliminary report on effects of photocoagulation therapy. *Am J Ophthalmol* **81**:383–396.

Chapter 7

OCULOPLASTICS

7.1 Eyelid Disorders

Learning Objectives
- Be aware of common causes of eyelid lumps and bumps and be alert to malignant lesions.
- Know how to classify ptosis based on onset and cause and understand the mechanism of ptosis.
- Be familiar with common eyelid malpositions including entropion and ectropion.
- Know how to evaluate a patient with eyelid injury and be familiar with principles of management.

Lumps and Bumps

Due to the unique anatomic features of the eyelid, lesions on the eyelid may have distinct presentations compared with similar lesions elsewhere in the body. Clinical judgment is important for identifying benign eyelid lesions while recognizing those with malignant potential that require biopsy.

Chalazion

- Chalazia typically appear as characteristically hard and usually painless (unless infected) lid nodules overlying the tarsus (Fig. 7.1)

- These growths occur due to obstruction of the orifices of the meibomian glands. Subsequently, the sebaceous contents of these glands are forced into the tarsus and surrounding soft tissues of the eyelid, leading to a chronic localised inflammatory response

- The classic histopathologic finding in chalazia is chronic lipogranulomatous inflammation

- Management: Most chalazia resolve by themselves within several days to weeks, but sometimes can take months to completely disappear. Medical therapy includes warm compresses, lid scrubs and antibiotic ointment. A large or persistent chalazion may require incision and curettage

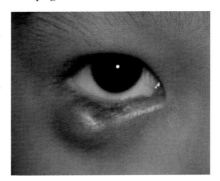

Fig. 7.1. A large lower lid chalazion with signs of inflammation.

Hordeolum

- This is an acute focal infection (usually staphylococcal) involving either the glands of Zeis (external hordeola) or, less frequently, the meibomian glands (internal hordeola)
- Medical therapy for hordeola includes eyelid hygiene (lid scrubs), warm compresses and topical antibiotic ointment. If an external hordeolum is centred around a lash follicle, the lash can be pulled to enhance drainage. Systemic antibiotics may be indicated if the hordeola is complicated by preseptal cellulitis. Internal hordeola may occasionally evolve into chalazia, which may require surgical incision and curettage

Benign and Premalignant Lesions

Embryologically, the skin and palpebral conjunctiva of the eyelid develop from the surface ectoderm, whereas the remaining structures originate from the mesoderm. Nearly all eyelid tumours arise from the epidermis, dermis, and adnexal structures. The adnexal structures include the sweat glands (glands of Moll), hair follicles, and sebaceous glands (Meibomian glands and glands of Zeis)

Table 7.1. Examples of Benign and Premalignant Eyelid Lesions Categorised according to their Layer of Origin

Layer	Lesions
Epidermis	Squamous cell papilloma, seborrheic keratosis, keratoacanthoma, actinic keratosis
Dermis	Nevus
Cystic lesions	Epidermal inclusion cyst, dermoid cyst
Sweat gland tumours	Hidrocystoma, syringoma
Hair follicle tumours	Pilomatrixoma, trichoepithelioma
Sebaceous gland tumors	Sebaceous adenoma

- Majority of tumours occurring on the eyelid are benign, a number of these lesions may be difficult to distinguish from malignant tumours based on clinical examination alone
- Typically, benign lesions do not ulcerate, bleed, or cause loss of lashes or destruction of normal eyelid architecture
- Atypical lesions may be more difficult to identify accurately. Histopathologic confirmation is necessary to establish a definitive diagnosis in some cases

Malignant Lesions

Skin cancers are one of the most common malignancies in the human body, with the eyelids being one of the frequent sites of involvement. There are geographic differences in the incidence of eyelid tumours as a result of skin type and sun exposure. In white populations, basal cell carcinoma (BCC) is the most frequent eyelid malignancy, followed by squamous cell carcinoma (SCC), sebaceous gland carcinoma (SGC), and melanoma. In more pigmented populations appendageal tumours such as SGC make up a greater proportion

Although each tumour has characteristic clinical features, there are certain signs that are suggestive of malignancy: loss of normal lid architecture, madarosis, tethering to deeper structures, and growth or change of a lesion's colour, border, or size

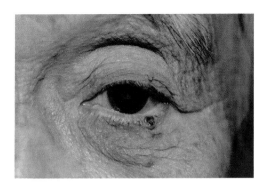

Fig. 7.2. Left lower lid pigmented BCC with rolled edges and an ulcerated crater in the centre.

Basal Cell Carcinoma

- Basal cell carcinoma (BCC) is one of the most common human malignancies
- Risk factors include ultraviolet (UV) light exposure, fair skin, immunosuppression, genetic disorders such as basal cell nevus syndrome (BCNS, Gorlin syndrome) and xeroderma pigmentosum
- BCC most commonly occurs on the lower eyelid, followed by the medial canthus, upper lid, and lateral canthus
- The following clinical presentations can occur:
  - Nodular: A pearly papule or nodule with surface telangiectasia and a rolled edge. It gradually enlarges to form a dome-shaped lesion, which may develop central ulceration
  - Superficial: A slow-growing, scaly, erythematous patch or plaque which may resemble dermatitis
  - Morpheic (sclerosing): An indurated, poorly defined, white to pink, scar-like plaque. This appearance is also sometimes termed "infiltrative" BCC
  - Pigmented (Fig. 7.2): BCC can have uniform or variegated brown, gray-blue, or black pigmentation and may mimic nevi or melanoma. This type is most common among pigmented races and is uncommon in whites
- Metastasis is rare in BCC
- Excision with confirmation of 3–4mm clear margins by histopathologic examination is the mainstay of treatment

Squamous Cell Carcinoma

- Squamous cell carcinoma (SCC) accounts for 5% to 10% of eyelid malignancies in whites but is rare in pigmented races
- Compared to BCC, it is a more aggressive tumour with a higher risk of perineural, nodal, and distant spread
- Risk factors include UVB radiation, pre-existing injured skin (e.g. ulcers, burns), immunosuppression, presence of precancerous lesions (e.g. actinic keratosis), genetic conditions (e.g. albinism, xeroderma pigmentosum)
- In the periocular area, they are most common on the lower lid, followed by the medial canthus, the upper lid, and the lateral canthus

- SCC has a wide range of clinical appearances
  - The majority are painless, scaling nodules or plaques with irregular rolled edges, fissuring, and ulceration
  - Others can form cutaneous horns, papillomas, or large fungating masses
- SCC can be neurotrophic when perineural invasion facilitates tumour spread into the orbit and cranial cavity
- Regional and distant metastatic spread occurs in 2% to 10% of periocular SCC
- Periocular SCC should be excised with intraoperative margin control, with either frozen section or Moh's micrographic surgery (MSS). A minimum 4mm margin has been advised for SCC

Sebaceous Gland Carcinoma

- Sebaceous gland carcinoma (SGC) can arise from the Meibomian glands, glands of Zeis, and sebaceous glands. They are most frequent in the eyelids because of the density of these glands. Other periocular sites include the eye-brow, caruncle, lacrimal gland and conjunctiva
- Reported risk factors for SGC include advanced age, Asian or South Asian race, women and previous irradiation to the head and neck
- SGC (Fig. 7.3) may masquerade not only as various inflammatory conditions such as blepharoconjunctivitis or chalazion but also as premalignant lesions and other benign or malignant tumours
  - The nodular form of SGC presents as a discrete, hard, immobile nodule commonly located in the upper tarsal plate having a yellowish appearance
  - The pagetoid variety of SGC occurs with intraepithelial infiltration of the lid margin and/or conjunctiva causing diffuse thickening and loss of eyelashes resembling chronic blepharoconjunctivitis
- Surgical excision, with 5-mm margins and margin control, is the recommended treatment. Orbital involvement usually necessitates exenteration, and nodal involvement is cleared with neck dissection. Adjunctive treatment (cryotherapy, radiotherapy and chemotherapy) may be used for advanced lesions or those with significant intraepithelial spread

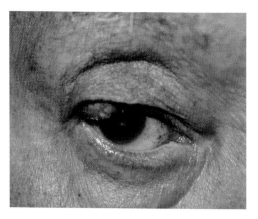

Fig. 7.3. Pigmented lesion on right upper lid margin with yellowish deposits suspicious of lipid and overlying telangiectasia with loss of lashes. Incisional biopsy confirmed SGC.

Ptosis

"Ptosis" refers to drooping or inferior displacement of any anatomical structure. "Blepharoptosis" (usually simply referred to as "ptosis") refers to drooping or inferior displacement of the upper eyelid

Ptosis can be classified by
- Onset
  - Congenital
  - Acquired
- Cause
  - Myogenic
  - Aponeurotic
  - Neurogenic
  - Mechanical
  - Traumatic

Anatomy and Function

The upper eyelid retractors comprise the following:
- Levator muscle
  - Primary retractor of upper eyelid
  - Supported at orbital aperture by Whitnall's ligament
  - Becomes collagenous aponeurosis that inserts on tarsal plate
- Muller's muscle
  - Responsible for involuntary upper eyelid elevation
- Frontalis muscle
  - Lifts brows
  - Weak retractor of upper eyelids

Evaluation

History

Pertinent points to ask in any patient with ptosis include:
- Medical history
  - Medication history: Anticoagulants
  - Previous eye or eyelid surgeries
  - Previous periorbital trauma
  - Onset and duration to distinguish congenital from acquired
  - Any variability in degree of ptosis during the day to rule out myasthenia-related ptosis
  - Complaints of diplopia
  - Dysphonia, dyspnea, dysphagia, proximal muscle weakness
  - Family history
  - How ptosis is affecting the patient's daily activities

Physical examination

A complete examination of any patient with ptosis includes:

- Vertical interpalpebral fissure height
  - Widest point between lower and upper eyelid
- Margin-reflex distance 1 (MRD-1)
  - Distance between upper eyelid margin and corneal light reflex in primary position
- Upper eyelid crease position
  - A high crease and deep superior sulcus is suggestive of aponeurotic ptosis
  - An absent or poorly formed lid crease is suggestive of congenital ptosis
- Levator function
  - Measuring eyelid excursion from downgaze to upgaze with frontalis muscle function negated
- Position of ptotic eyelid in downgaze
  - Congenital ptosis: eyelid higher in downgaze than contralateral side
  - Involutional ptosis: eyelid ptotic in all positions of gaze; usually worsens in downgaze
- Visual function and refractive error
  - Congenital or childhood ptosis: amblyopia occurs in approximately 20% of congenital ptosis
- Extraocular movements
- Extraocular muscle dysfunction associated with ptosis in various conditions
  - Oculomotor palsy
  - Ocular myasthenia gravis (MG)
  - Chronic progressive external ophthalmoplegia (CPEO)
- Pupils
  - Horner syndrome – miosis
  - CN 3 palsy – mydriasis
- Head position, chin elevation, brow position, brow action in attempted upgaze
- Tear film, lagophthalmos, Bell's reflex, corneal sensation
  - To identify factors which may predispose patient to complications of ptosis repair such as dryness and keratopathy
- Synkinesis
  - Marcus Gunn jaw-winking ptosis
  - Aberrant regeneration of 3rd or 7th CN palsy

Acquired Aponeurotic Ptosis

- Most common of all forms of ptosis
- Due to stretching or dehiscence of levator aponeurosis / Disinsertion of levator aponeurosis from normal position
- Common causes
  - Senile changes of the levator aponeurosis and its insertion onto the tarsus
  - Frequent eye rubbing

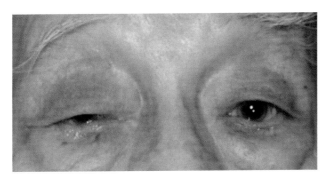

Fig. 7.4. Patient with right sided aponeurotic ptosis causing obstruction of visual axis.

- Contact lens wear
- Previous intraocular surgery
- Characteristics (Fig. 7.4)
  - High or absent eyelid crease
  - Deep superior sulcus
  - Levator function may vary but usually fair to good
  - Ptosis may worsen in downgaze

Congenital Myogenic Ptosis

- In most cases of congenital myogenic ptosis, the cause is idiopathic.
  - Rarely it may be associated with a genetic dysmorphic syndrome such as blepharophimosis syndrome.
- Histologically, the levator muscles of patients with congenital ptosis are dystrophic. The levator muscle and aponeurotic tissues appear to be infiltrated with fat and fibrous tissue.
- Although not all patients with congenital ptosis need surgical intervention, patients need to be closely monitored for the possible development of amblyopia from visual deprivation or uncorrected astigmatism.
- Characteristics (Fig. 7.5)
  - Decreased levator function, usually poor
  - Eyelid lag on downgaze
  - Lagophthalmos (sometimes)
  - Absent or poorly formed lid crease

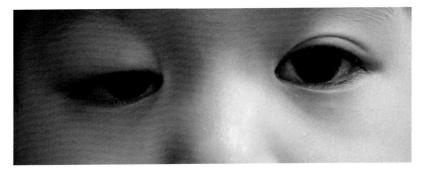

Fig. 7.5. Child with right congenital myogenic ptosis. Note the absent lid crease.

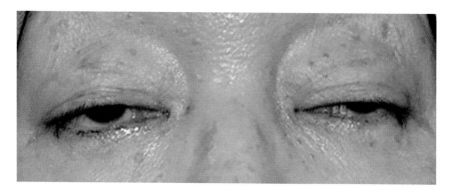

Fig. 7.6. Patient with myogenic ptosis with ophthalmolplegia secondary to CPEO.

Myogenic Ptosis

- Other than congenital myogenic ptosis, causes of myogenic ptosis include CPEO (Fig. 7.6), myotonic dystrophy, oculopharyngeal muscular dystrophy
- **Myasthenia gravis** (MG) may be included in both the neurogenic and myogenic classifications (See Chapter 9 Neuro-ophthalmology)

Neurogenic Ptosis

- Causes
  - Dysfunction of the oculomotor nerve (aetiologies include vascular, ischaemic, demyelination, tumours and trauma)
  - Dysfunction of sympathetic innervation to Mullers muscle (Horner's syndrome)
  - Synkinetic ptosis such as Marcus Gunn jaw winking syndrome
- In cases of neurogenic ptosis due to dysfunction of the oculomotor nerve, there is innervational deficiency in levator muscle function
  - There may be associated neurologic findings
  - Surgical correction of ptosis should be deferred until its cause has been thoroughly investigated and the condition has stabilised
  - The ocular misalignment must be addressed before ptosis correction
  - Levator function will remain defective despite reestablishment of adequate eyelid height

Treatment of Ptosis

- Non-surgical treatment
  - Eyelid crutches attached to eyeglass frames
  - Taping of upper lid
- Surgical treatment
  - Usually done under local anesthesia (except children)
  - Three broad categories:
    i. External/Transcutaneous/Anterior: Levator repair/resection
    - Skin incision
    - Tightening levator muscle to elevate eyelid
    - Reserved for fair to good levator function, although maximal levator resection can be attempted for poor levator function

  ii. Internal/Transconjunctival/Posterior: Conjunctivomullerectomy

- No skin incision
- Surgery on Mullers muscle from conjunctival approach
- Usually for mild (2mm or less) ptosis with positive phenylephrine test

  iii. Frontalis muscle suspension

- Brow suspension
- For patients with poor to absent levator function
- Materials for brow suspension include autogenous or preserved fascia lata, silicon rods, monofilament nylon, braided polyester, etc.

Eyelid Malpositions

Entropion

Entropion is an eyelid malposition resulting in inward turning of the eyelid margin (Fig. 7.7). This causes the myocutaneous border of the eyelid and lashes to be directed towards the globe, resulting in conjunctival irritation and corneal abrasion

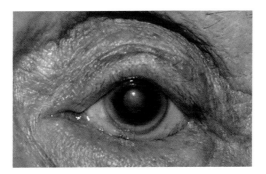

Fig. 7.7. Left lower lid involutional entropion. Note the inward rolling of the eyelid margin with lashes buried and touching the conjunctiva.

Classification

The pathophysiology depends on the type of entropion:

- Acute spastic
  - Following ocular inflammation/irritation
  - Sustained orbicularis contraction > inward rotation of eyelid margin
- Involutional
  - Weakness of inferior retractors
  - Horizontal lid laxity
  - Overriding of preseptal to pretarsal orbicularis oculi
  - Tarsal plate atrophy
- Cicatricial
  - Caused by vertical tarsoconjunctival contracture and internal rotation of eyelid margin
    i. Autoimmune: ocular cicatricial pemphigoid (OCP)
    ii. Inflammation: chronic meibomitis, Stevens Johnson syndrome (SJS)

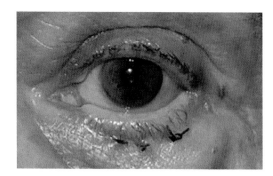

Fig. 7.8. Left lower lid entropion treated with Quickert sutures to rotate the eyelid margin outwards.

iii. Infection: trachoma, herpes zoster (HZ)

iv. Surgery, trauma

Management

Medical therapy may be warranted for patients who decline surgery and as a temporizing manoeuvre in patients who may improve spontaneously

- Topical lubricants are helpful for protecting the ocular surface and may break the cycle in patients with spastic entropion due to dry eye syndrome
- Treatment of blepharitis may help alleviate spastic entropion
- Small amounts of botulinum toxin (BOTOX®) may be effective for spastic entropion by weakening the pretarsal orbicularis oculi muscle
- Treat underlying cause of cicatricial entropion, e.g. OCP and SJS

Multiple surgical procedures have been described for the management of entropion. The surgical correction must be directed at repair of the primary anatomic defects

- For instance, in involutional entropion, both inferior retractor repair and horizontal lid shortening (e.g. lateral tarsal strip) are usually required to address inferior retractor weakness and horizontal lid laxity respectively
- A less satisfactory and temporary procedure is the placement of full thickness Quickert-Rathbun type sutures to rotate the eyelid margin outwards (Fig. 7.8)

Ectropion

Ectropion is an eyelid malposition resulting in outward turning of the eyelid margin. This leads to lagophthalmos, inadequate corneal protection, discomfort, and ultimately epithelial and stromal injury. Tear drainage dysfunction results from poor apposition of the puncta to the globe. The causes are varied, and correction must be directed at the source of the pathologic process

Classification

Ectropion can be classified by the cause:

- Involutional
  - Horizontal lid laxity + dehiscence of lower lid retractors
- Paralytic
  - Facial palsy (Fig. 7.9)
    i. Loss of orbicularis tone results in outward displacement of lower lid under influence of gravity

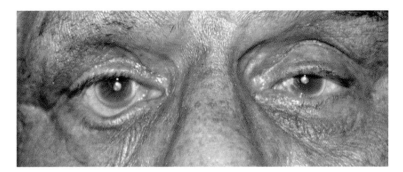

Fig. 7.9. Right lower lid paralytic ectropion secondary to lower motor neuron facial palsy. He had concurrent brow ptosis as well, and had shaved his eyebrow to avoid the hairs from the eyebrow causing irritation to his eye.

     ii. Paralytic ectropion often associated with brow ptosis and secondary dermatochalasis.
- Cicatricial
  - Loss of skin
    - i. Chemical/thermal burns
    - ii. Trauma (mechanical/surgical)
  - Chronic inflammation of eyelid
    - i. Rosacea
    - ii. Atopic dermatitis
    - iii. HZ infection
- Mechanical
  - Mass effect induced by bulk tumours of eyelid

Management

Management is directed at the underlying cause
- In involutional ectropion, repair is directed at tightening the lax components of eyelid structure. The most common and useful lid shortening procedure is the lateral tarsal strip procedure
- In paralytic ectropion secondary to facial nerve palsy, the goal in management is to protect the cornea. It is important to determine the likelihood of facial palsy recovery before offering more permanent surgical procedures. Surgical procedures for facial palsy are varied and include tarsorrhaphy, lateral tarsal strip, medial and lateral canthoplasty, mid-face lift, and direct brow lift

Eyelid Injuries

Head and facial injuries frequently involve the periocular area and can cause significant morbidity

Initial Assessment

- When evaluating a patient who has sustained any type of trauma, life-threatening injuries should first be addressed or ruled out before assessing for ocular and adnexal trauma
- In the setting of trauma, the physician should not forget the basics of life support (airway, breathing, circulation) and systemic trauma assessments

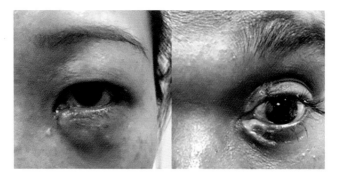

Fig. 7.10. Small lacerations in medial aspect of lower lid in different patients. Probing confirmed laceration of lower canaliculus.

History

- Evaluation should begin with a complete history
- This includes the medical, ocular, and surgical history and pointed questions about the injury
- The mechanism, timing, and location of the injury should be recorded
- Tetanus status and any changes in the patient's vision or facial sensation should be noted
- The patient's allergies and last oral intake are important, and the patient should not be allowed to eat or drink until the evaluation and any surgical planning is complete

Examination

A full examination for any lid and adnexal trauma includes the following:
- Visual acuity
- Pupils
- Extraocular motility
- Eyelids
  - Any lacerations should be noted, including the location and depth
  - Fat protrusion through the eyelid is an indication of orbital septum penetration and requires ophthalmologic consultation before exploration and repair
- Canaliculi and lacrimal system
  - Eyelid lacerations medials to the puncta are assumed to involve the canaliculus (canaliculi) until proven otherwise (Fig. 7.10)
- Orbit (refer to Chapter 7.2 on "Orbital Trauma")

General Principles of Repair for Eyelid Lacerations

- Clean wound and remove foreign body if any
- Careful handling of tissues
- Careful alignment of anatomy
  - Lid margin, lash line, grey line, etc.
  - Lid margin lacerations usually repaired prior to extramarginal lacerations for better anatomical realignment
- Close in layers

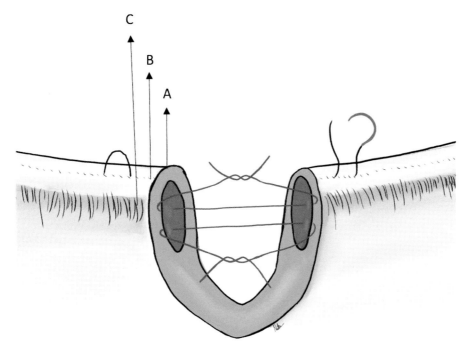

Fig. 7.11. Sutures placed at the tarsus, and lid margin.

- Timing
  - Ideally within 12–24 hours of injury, but can be delayed based on patient factors

Eyelid Margin Lacerations

- Carefully align lid margin with 6/0 silk suture to prevent notching
- Close tarsal plate with 6/0 Vicryl (partial thickness of tarsus)
- Additional margin silk sutures (Fig. 7.11)
  - Mucocutaneous junction (A)
  - Gray line (B)
  - Lash line (C)

Take home messages

- Although most eyelid tumours are benign, some are clinically difficult to distinguish from malignant tumours and may require a biopsy.
- Common malignant tumours of the eyelid are basal cell carcinoma (BCC), squamous cell carcinoma (SCC).
- Aponeurotic ptosis is the most common cause of adult-acquired ptosis whereas the most common myogenic ptosis is congenital in origin.
- Entropion and ectropion are common malpositions of the eyelid and correction must be directed at the source of the pathologic process.
- General principles for repair of eyelid lacerations include careful handling of tissues, proper alignment of anatomy especially for lid margin lacerations.

7.2 Orbital Disorders

Learning Objectives

- Know how to differentiate preseptal from orbital cellulitis and be familiar with their management.
- Be familiar with the signs and symptoms of thyroid eye disease (TED) and various sight threatening complications.
- Understand the management principles of TED.
- Be aware of common orbital tumours and how they may present.
- Know how to assess a patient with trauma and what to look out for in a patient with suspected orbital fractures.

Orbital Cellulitis

Orbital cellulitis is one of the life-threatening ophthalmic conditions. It is considered on same spectrum of disease with preseptal cellulitis, however the distinction between these two conditions is important.

Orbital cellulitis is the infection of the ocular adnexal tissue posterior to the orbital septum while preseptal cellulitis is infection that only involves structures anterior to the septum, such as eyelid tissue. The septum is a layer of fascia extending superiorly from the orbital rim to the levator aponeurosis in the upper eyelid, as well as to the inferior border of the tarsus in the lower eyelid. In orbital cellulitis, the infection could spread posteriorly, causing cavernous sinus thrombosis as well as intracranial involvement, resulting in morbidity and mortality.

Chandler's Classification

It describes the level of involvement of the cellulitis. Although this suggests a sequential progression, any infection may involve one or more stage and progress in either direction, so its usefulness is debated

Stage 1: Preseptal cellulitis
Stage 2: Orbital cellulitis
Stage 3: Subperiosteal abscess
Stage 4: Orbital abscess
Stage 5: Cavernous sinus thrombosis

Aetiology

- Adjacent infection in surrounding structures
  - Sinusitis
  - Eyelids (including hordeola)
  - Lacrimal sac
  - Dental infections
- External causes
  - Trauma
  - Surgery
- Endogenous causes (bacteraemia)
- Ophthalmic causes (e.g. endophthalmitis with extraocular extension)

Pathogens

The pathogens involved depend on source and patient age

- *Staph. aureus* and streptococcal species (including pneumococcus) are associated with eyelid and lacrimal sac infections
- Community-acquired MRSA is increasing in incidence in some regions and may penetrate small breaks in the skin
- In the past, *H. influenza* was a common organism in young children with dacryocystitis or hematogenous sources but is rare in regions where HiB vaccination is available
- Sinus infections
  - In children under 9-years of age: commonly caused by a single aerobic non-spore-forming bacteria
  - In adolescents and, particularly, adults: more likely to be polymicrobial and to include facultative anaerobes
- Penetrating trauma with organic foreign bodies may introduce fungi, especially aspergillus

History

Preseptal Cellulitis

- Pain of the eyelid/periorbital tissues
- Eyelid redness and swelling

Orbital Cellulitis

- Symptoms of preseptal cellulitis, as well as:
- Blurring of vision
- Swelling and injection of conjunctiva
- Double vision
- Pain on eye movements
- Systemic symptoms such as fever

Other Relevant History that should be Sought

- Symptoms of sinusitis (facial pain, post-nasal drip, etc.)
- Trauma
- Insect bites
- Immunocompromised status (uncontrolled diabetes, malignancies, etc.)

Examination

A full examination for peri-orbital cellulitis includes the following:

- Optic nerve function
  - Visual acuity
  - Colour vision (Ishihara, D-15 charting)
  - Pupils (RAPD)
  - Visual fields (by confrontation)
  - Examination of the optic disc (for disc swelling)

- Chemosis
- Ocular motility (looking for limitation)
- Proptosis
  - Using an exophthalmometer if possible
  - If not available, this can be grossly observed from looking down from above the patient's head to observe protrusion of the corneal apex on the affected side
- Systemic evaluation, e.g. for fever and toxicity

Investigations

- Blood cultures before starting IV antibiotics
- Swab culture of purulent material (e.g. cutaneous wounds, nasal secretions, or conjunctival discharge)
- High resolution computed tomography (Fig. 7.12) scanning is helpful to assess the severity of the infection, look for sinus disease, and complications such as subperiosteal abscess and cavernous sinus thrombosis.

Management of Orbital Cellulitis

- Patients with orbital cellulitis should be admitted for treatment and close monitoring.
- Systemic antibiotics should be instituted early and not delayed while waiting for imaging studies.
- Indications for surgery:
  - Progressive disease despite antibiotic use
  - Decrease in vision
  - Subperiosteal or orbital abscesses causing visual compromise, or large abscesses especially in older patients > 9 years
  - Invasive fungal disease (e.g. mucormycosis)
- Referral to otolaryngologist if sinus disease is detected

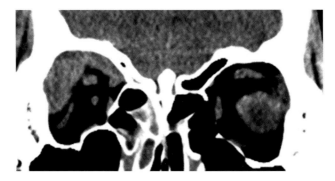

Fig. 7.12. Right superior subperiosteal abscesses in a patient with orbital cellulitis.

Thyroid Eye Disease

Thyroid eye disease (TED), also known as thyroid-associated orbitopathy (TAO) or Graves orbitopathy (GO), is a tissue specific autoimmune orbito-facial inflammatory disorder. It is one of most challenging syndromes to manage owing to its complex and poorly understood pathogenesis.

What is Thyroid Eye Disease and Why does it Happen?

- Thyroid eye disease (TED) is an autoimmune disease. It is mainly associated with an over-active thyroid due to Graves' disease, although it does sometimes occur in people with an under-active or normally functioning thyroid.

- The eyes are particularly vulnerable to Graves' eye disease, because the autoimmune attack often targets the eye muscles and connective tissue within the orbital socket. This likely occurs because the tissues within the orbit contain proteins that appear similar to the immune system as those of the thyroid gland.

- As a result of the autoimmune attack, the eye muscles and fatty tissue behind the eye become inflamed. This can cause the eyes to be pushed forward and the eyelids to be pulled upwards to some degree, giving rise to "staring" or "bulging" eyes. In the active state, the eyes feel painful and tight, and the eyes and eyelids often become swollen and red (Fig. 7.13).

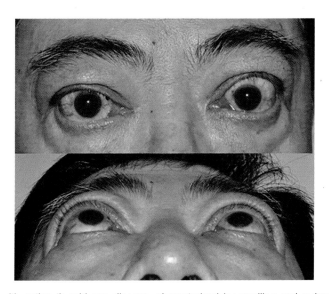

Fig. 7.13. Patient with active thyroid eye disease, characterised by swelling and redness of the upper and lower lids, conjunctival redness, swelling of the curuncle and orbital pain. This patient also has lid retraction and proptosis of both eyes.

- In the inactive or chronic phase, the extraocular muscles may become swollen and stiff, resulting in double vision. Rarely, TED can cause blindness from pressure on the optic nerve (compressive neuropathy) or exposure keratopathy.

- Apart from activity, TED is also classified based on severity (mild, moderate or severe).
  - In mild cases of TED, patients may only complain of sensitive and dry eyes, associated with increased tearing. Some mild cases may have associated lid signs, namely lid retraction and lid lag.
  - In moderate TED, the patient usually has worsening of soft tissue signs, with greater lid retraction and exophthalmos. The patient may also experience diplopia (double vision) outside 30° of primary gaze.
  - In severe TED (Fig. 7.14), the patient may experience severe exposure keratopathy not amenable to conservative management, compressive optic neuropathy, or diplopia in primary gaze, or within 30° of primary gaze.

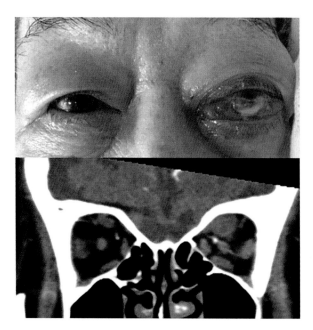

Fig. 7.14. Patient with severe active thyroid eye disease. This lady had an active flare of the disease with progressive proptosis resulting in exposure keratopathy and a resultant corneal ulcer. Corresponding computed tomography (CT) scan of the orbits show enlargement and crowding of the extraocular muscles around the optic nerve in the left orbit.

What can be Done for Thyroid Eye Disease?

- For all patients with TED, the following measures may prevent the disease progression:
  - Symptomatic treatment of dry eyes including topical lubricants, sunglasses in bright sunlight or temporary punctal plugs.
  - Give up smoking, both active and passive, in order to reduce the severity, duration of activity, degree of scarring, and risk of optic nerve involvement.
  - Co-manage all patients with an endocrinologist, and ensure their thyroid disease is well-controlled at each visit.
- Classifying the patient into active or inactive disease is very important from management point of view.
  - Active disease requires immunosuppression, of which intravenous methylprednisolone is the treatment of choice.
  - Steroid sparing immunosuppressant therapy, given in collaboration with the Rheumatology team, is considered for their steroid sparing effects especially in cases of persistent inflammation.
  - External beam radiotherapy, given by radiation oncologists, may also be considered in those patients who have contraindications or intolerance to various forms of corticosteroid/steroid sparing agents, but generally avoided both in the young and the elderly, as well as those with diabetes.
- Surgical management for TED includes the following:
  - Orbital decompression and this may be done for several indications
    - i. Proptosis
    - ii. Persistent congestion after immunosuppression

iii. Compressive optic neuropathy

iv. As a staging procedure, in preparation for strabismus or eyelid surgery

- Strabismus surgery: Surgery on the extraocular muscles is performed to correct the misalignment of the eyes.
- Eyelid surgery and these include surgery to correct
    i. Upper or lower lid retraction
    ii. Upper or lower blepharoplasty (to remove excess skin and fat)

Conclusion

Thyroid eye disease remains a major clinical and therapeutic challenge. It has been shown to have a negative impact on psychosocial functioning and quality of life, even in mild cases. Fortunately, there are continued advances in the understanding of pathogenesis, and risk-benefit profile of various medical and surgical interventions, making it a much more manageable disease compared to decades ago. The ultimate goal is early identification of TED, with effective halting and reversal of the active inflammatory process. The need for a patient-centered, multidisciplinary approach to these patients is important, to ensure careful and coordinated care for these patients.

Orbital Tumours

Orbital Tumours

- The orbit is the bony socket in which the eye is located. It consists of a floor, roof and walls on either side.
- It is possible for tumours to form in this space, between the eye and the bones.
- These tumours range in seriousness, from benign lumps that can be observed, to malignant tumours that require complex treatment regimens.
- Tumours can be congenital or acquired.
- They may involve other areas outside the orbit, including the sinuses or even the brain.
- Orbital tumours may arise from any of the tissue types that are normally found in the orbit, including blood vessels, nervous tissue, bone and lymphoid tissue.

Presentation

- A tumour in the orbit may initially cause fullness in the area around the eye or it may cause proptosis.
- Patient may complain of double vision when the globe is moved significantly away from its normal position.
- Certain tumours can also affect the nerves in the area and cause pain.

Capillary Hemangioma

This is the most common tumour of the orbit in childhood. It is a vascular tumour, comprising of a series of anastomosing small vascular channels. A range of presentations exists, from a small lesion away from the eye, to a large lesion involving the eyelid and obstructing the visual axis of one of the eyes. The most concerning feature to the ophthalmologist is the proximity of involvement to the eye. Lesions of the eyelid can cause astigmatism (and possible resultant refractive amblyopia) from external pressure on the eye, as well as deprivational amblyopia if the visual axis is obstructed.

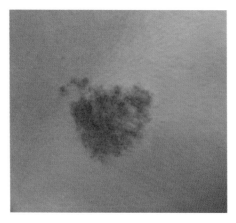

Fig. 7.15. Superficial capillary hemangioma (also known as strawberry nevus) appears as a raised, red, lumpy area of flesh anywhere on the body, including the head and neck.

Presentation

- This tumour often presents in the first few weeks of life, with typical enlargement in size up to the age of 2 years with subsequent reduction in size.
- 70% of lesions tend to regress by 7 years of age.

Clinical Appearance

- The tumour appears bright red when superficially located (earning the name "strawberry nevus") (Fig. 7.15).
- Deep tumours may cause a unilateral proptosis without any discoloration of the skin.

Management

- Indications for treatment
  - Amblyopia due to astigmatism or obstruction of visual axis
  - Optic nerve compression
  - Exposure keratopathy
- Treatment modalities
  - Beta-blockers
    - i. Topical
    - ii. Systemic: Propranolol is an effective medication and the main stay of treatment for capillary hemangiomas
  - Steroids
    - i. Local injection (only for superficial lesions)
    - ii. Systemic
  - Surgical resection
    - i. This is a last resort option as it is often difficult to remove the tumour while preserving normal anatomy.
  - Laser treatments
    - – can sometimes be used on superficial hemangiomas to prevent growth, diminish their size, or lighten their colour.

Cavernous Hemangioma

Cavernous hemangioma is the old term for what is now classified as a venous malformation. It is a tumour that consists of a collection of vascular channels and is most common benign orbital tumour in adults. It affects females more than males. Mean age of presentation is in the 4th to 5th decade of life. It often results in a tumour within the muscle cone that causes a unilateral axial proptosis. However, some cases are discovered incidentally on radiographic imaging studies.

History
- Duration of proptosis
- Diplopia
- Blurring of vision

Examination
- Visual acuity, intraocular pressure
- Ocular motility
- Exophthalmometry
- Complete ocular examination, looking for choroidal folds due to compression

Investigations
- Computed tomography scan of the orbits (Fig. 7.16) shows a well-circumscribed round lesion with contrast enhancement

Treatment Options
- Observation: for asymptomatic tumours not causing proptosis or disfigurement
- Surgical resection: for tumours causing proptosis, diplopia, disfigurement or optic nerve compression.

Optic Nerve Glioma

Optic nerve glioma is a slow growing tumour of neural tissue origin that typically affects young children. 30% of affected children have Neurofibromatosis Type 1. The typical age of presentation is during the first decade of life.

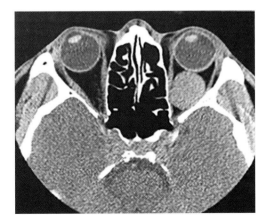

Fig. 7.16. CT showing a well-circumscribed intraconal mass in the left orbit. The mass was surgically excised and proven to be cavernous hemangioma.

Clinical Presentation

- Slow onset of visual loss
- Proptosis
- Fundoscopy shows optic disc swelling, then pallor
- Chiasmal and intracranial spread is possible

Investigations

- Computed tomography scanning shows a fusiform enlargement of the optic nerve
- MRI may be useful to evaluate any suspected intracranial involvement

Management

- Small tumours with minimal visual compromise can be observed
- Surgical excision is indicated if there is poor visual or very significant proptosis
- Radiotherapy may be considered for tumours with intracranial involvement which are not suitable for resection

Optic Nerve Sheath Meningioma

Optic nerve sheath meningiomas (ONSM) arise from the meningoepithelial tissues around the optic nerve. They are typically slow growing tumours, affecting middle-aged women most commonly.

Clinical Features

- Gradual impairment of vision
- Gradual proptosis
- May present with optociliary shunts and optic nerve atrophy

Investigations

- CT shows thickening and calcification of the optic nerve.
- MRI studies with gadolinium contrast as well as fat suppression are ideal for evaluating ONSM. MRI will again demonstrate diffuse, tubular thickening of the optic nerve sheath encasing the optic nerve, often producing a characteristic "tram track" sign on axial cuts or a "doughnut" sign on coronal cuts. The tumour enhances with contrast infusion. MRI is particularly useful for delineating the extent of the tumour and for evaluating for intracranial extension.

Management

- Small tumours with minimal visual compromise can be observed
- Surgical excision is indicated if there is poor visual or very significant proptosis
- Radiotherapy may be considered for tumours with intracranial involvement which are not suitable for resection

Orbital Metastases

Orbital metastases are not a common cause of proptosis, and are less common as compared to choroidal metastases. However, the ophthalmologist may be the first doctor to detect the presence of a malignancy. The most common metastases in adults are from breast, bronchus, prostate, skin, gastrointestinal tract and the kidney.

Rhabdomyosarcoma

Rhabdomyosarcoma is the commonest primary orbital malignant tumour in children. It is comprised of poorly differentiated mesenchymal cells, which possess the potential to differentiate into striated muscle. It is an aggressive tumour that requires prompt recognition as it may masquerade as an orbital cellulitis.

Clinical Features

- Typical presentation is during the first decade of life
- Rapid onset of unilateral proptosis that is progressive
- Swelling and redness of overlying skin
- Ptosis and strabismus may be present
- Skin is not warm to the touch, unlike orbital cellulitis
- May masquerade as an orbital inflammation or orbital cellulitis

Imaging Findings

- CT and MRI scanning usually shows an ill-defined mass
- There are often areas of bony destruction

Management

- An urgent workup is required for these patients
- Biopsy of the tissue is required for histological diagnosis
- Surgical debulking may improve staging and tumour response to treatment
- Radiotherapy and chemotherapy are options for tumours not amenable to surgery
- Exenteration is reserved for recurrent disease and carries significant morbidity

General Principles of Management for Orbital Tumours

Often a multi-disciplinary team is required, including adult or paediatric oncologists, radiation oncologists, social workers, prosthetics specialists, geneticists and the ophthalmologist.

- Imaging with CT or MRI scan of the orbits and/or brain is required.
  - CT is better than MRI for bone definition
  - MRI is better than CT for soft tissue definition
- Tissue diagnosis via biopsy or other tissue sampling method may be required.
- This will be sent to a specialised laboratory to be analysed by a pathologist trained in ocular oncology.
- Based on the tissue diagnosis and further ancillary tests including tissue genetic or biochemical analysis, the ideal mode of therapy is decided, after consideration of multiple factors including:
  - The degree of systemic involvement
  - The aggressiveness of the tumour
  - The health of the patient
  - The wishes of the patient and family
  - The likely success rates of treatment

Orbital Trauma

Head and facial injuries frequently involve the periocular area and can cause significant morbidity.

Initial Assessment

- When evaluating a patient who has sustained any type of trauma, life-threatening injuries should first be addressed or ruled out before assessing for ocular and adnexal trauma.
- In the setting of trauma, the physician should not forget the basics of life support (airway, breathing, circulation) and systemic trauma assessments.

Orbital Fractures

Orbital wall fractures are commonly encountered in facial trauma. In more than 40% of all facial fractures, parts of the orbital rim and/or the internal orbit are injured showing various fracture patterns.

- The very anatomy of the orbit makes it prone to fractures, and it is therefore involved in a majority of midfacial fractures. However, just as the bony orbit protects the globe normally, the bony orbit gives way at its weak points to protect the globe when traumatised. Hence fractures are in fact a protective mechanism to the eye in times of trauma.

Typical Signs Pointing towards Orbital Fracture

- History of blunt trauma to face
- Periocular ecchymosis and oedema
- Enophthalmos (later sequelae)
- Infraorbital hypoaesthesia
- Ocular motility limitation; diplopia
- Hypoglobus
  - Severe orbital floor disruption
  - Roof fracture with superior orbital hematoma

Orbital Blow-out Fracture

- The orbital floor medial to the infraorbital groove, and the lamina papyracea overlying the ethmoidal sinuses, are relatively thin and may buckle and fracture when blunt force impacts the orbital soft tissue and bone margins causing a sudden rise in hydraulic pressure and buckling of the thinner bone. This gives rise to orbital floor and medial wall blow out fractures respectively (Figs. 7.17 and 7.18).

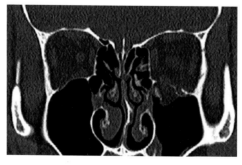

Fig. 7.17. Left orbital floor blow-out fracture, medial to infraorbital groove with mild herniation of orbital contents into maxillary sinus. The inferior rectus is not entrapped.

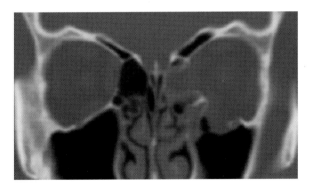

Fig. 7.18. Large blow-out fractures of the left orbital floor and medial wall, with herniation of the medial and inferior recti into the adjacent sinuses, along with the orbital contents.

- Orbital tissue herniating into the sinus through the resulting defect in the orbital floor may become entrapped, causing diplopia, and if the displacement of the bony fragment is large enough, enophthalmos may develop.
- Two theories have been proposed — the "buckling" theory and "hydraulic" theory.
  - In the former, blowout fractures are believed to occur through force transmission from the more rigid infraorbital rim to the relatively weak orbital floor. Blunt trauma to the face causes the pressure wave to travel posteriorly, acutely compressing the bones of the orbit in the anterior-posterior direction. This increase in bony pressure causes the weakest point in the orbit to "buckle" and crack, with the bone fragment pushed inferiorly.
  - In the "hydraulic" theory, the eyeball, when struck directly by an object such as a fist or a baseball, is thrust posteriorly, transiently raising the pressure within the orbit. As the intraorbital pressure increases dramatically and suddenly, the floor of the orbit "blows out" inferiorly at the point of greatest weakness. Hence, the hydraulic pressure from the globe is transmitted to the bony orbit, resulting in fracture of the thin medial orbital floor.

Trapdoor Fracture

- A "trapdoor" orbital fracture is an isolated orbital floor fracture which occurs when a bony fragment, often hinged medially, is transiently displaced inferiorly, allowing herniation of orbital contents into the maxillary sinus, which are then entrapped as the bony fragment returns toward its initial position (Fig. 7.18).
- It is postulated that before puberty, a large portion of the orbital floor consists of immature bone and overlies a small maxillary sinus. Hence, the bony floor in children and adolescents is relatively pliable, so that even minimal force can result in a small fracture segment swinging down and snapping back, thereby incarcerating orbital tissue.
- Despite severe limitation of ocular motility, orbital oedema or sign of soft tissue injury is relatively minimal. Hence it has also been termed as "the white-eyed blowout fracture" (Fig. 7.19). Such fractures are often associated with nausea and vomiting. An oculocardiac reflex can also occur manifesting in bradycardia especially on eliciting eye movements.

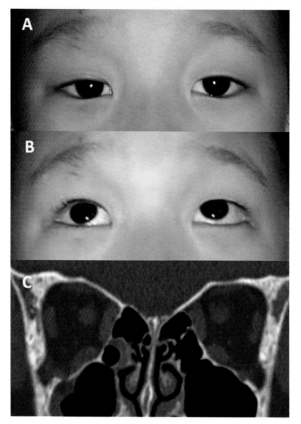

Fig. 7.19. (A) Five-year old boy who fell and hit his right eye. On examination, the eye is white without much periorbital oedema and ecchymosis. (B) There is limitation of the right eye on upgaze, raising the clinical suspicion of a trapdoor fracture. (C) On imaging, the fracture may be easily missed as the bony fragment has "snapped back" into position, incarcerating some orbital soft tissue.

Take home messages

- Orbital cellulitis can be life-threatening and treatment must be initiated promptly.
- Three questions to ask when assessing a patient with thyroid eye disease:
  - Is this thyroid eye disease?
  - Is it mild, moderate or severe?
  - Is it active or quiescent?
- Orbital tumours can arise from many structures including blood vessels, nervous tissue, bone and lymphoid tissue.
- Principles of management of orbital tumors include assessing the extent of involvement, establishing a tissue diagnosis and starting specific treatment.
- The most common sites of orbital fractures are the medial part of the orbital floor and medial wall.
- Trapdoor fracture should be suspected in any child with blunt trauma.

7.3 Lacrimal Disorders

Learning Objectives
Be aware of symptoms and signs of nasolacrimal duct obstruction in adults and children.

Acquired Nasolacrimal Duct Obstruction

Tears play a critical role in providing nutrients and protection to the cornea, in creating a smooth surface for clarity and in conveying emotions. There are three phases in normal tear flow: 1) production (lacrimal secretion, release of mucin from goblet cells and lipid from Meibomian glands), 2) distribution through eyelid blinking and the lacrimal pump, and 3) tear elimination through excretion and evaporation. Disorders in the lacrimal system may arise in any one of these three phases and require specific tests for confirmation and directed management dependent on the structures affected.

Obstruction of the drainage system can be congenital or acquired, and may result in persistent epiphora and mucopurulent discharge.

What is the Anatomy of the Lacrimal Drainage System? (Fig. 7.20)

- The lacrimal system consists of
  - **Puncta**: These are small openings of 0.2–0.3 mm diameter in the medial aspect of the upper and lower lid margin. Each punctum lies on the lacrimal papilla. The inferior punctum lies in apposition to the tear meniscus.
  - **Canaliculi**: Vertical canaliculi is 2 mm and horizontal canaliculi is 8 mm in length. They are 1 to 1.5 mm in diameter. Both the upper and lower canaliculi join to form the common canaliculus.
  - **Lacrimal Sac**: The common canaliculus then leads to the lacrimal sac. The lacrimal sac lies in the lacrimal sac fossa, which is bounded by the anterior and posterior lacrimal crests. The floor of the fossa comprises of the maxillary bone anteriorly and the lacrimal bone posteriorly.

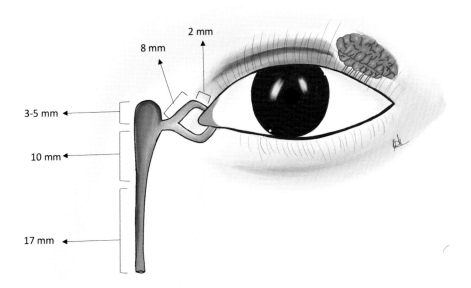

Fig. 7.20. Normal lacrimal drainage pathway.

- **Nasolacrimal duct**: The nasolacrimal duct lies within a bony canal which is 12 mm long, 3–5 mm wide. It passes down posteriorly at a 15-30° angle to open in the inferior meatus within the nasal cavity.

Clinical Features

- Epiphora
- Ocular discharge
- Sometimes lacrimal sac inflammation (dacryocystitis)

What is the Management of Nasolacrimal Duct Obstruction?

- In acute or chronic dacryocystitis (Fig. 7.21)
  - Topical and systemic antibiotics
  - Some surgeons believe in percutaneous drainage of lacrimal sac abscess
  - Dacryocystorhinostomy (DCR) is usually performed subsequently
- More recently, endoscopic lacrimal ductal recanalisation (ELDR) has been gaining popularity in treating partial or complete nasolacrimal duct obstructions.

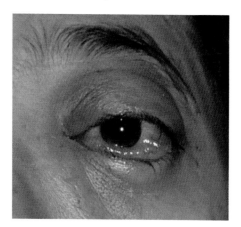

Fig. 7.21. Left acute dacryocystitis with erythema and swelling over the lacrimal sac region, chemosis, tearing and ocular discharge.

What is a Dacryocystorhinostomy?

- A dacryocystorhinostomy (DCR) is a procedure performed for the treatment of tearing (epiphora) due to blockage of the nasolacrimal duct.
- It creates an ostium between the tear sac and the nasal cavity by removing the mucosa and bone layers between them.
- There are two main approaches: External and Endoscopic
  - The external approach requires a skin incision.
  - The endoscopic approach creates the ostium from within the nose without the need for a skin incision.
  - Both have similar success rates, with their own advantages and disadvantages.

Congenital Nasolacrimal Duct Obstruction

Congenital nasolacrimal duct obstruction (NLDO) is a common condition that may affect up to 50% of newborns. It is caused by a membranous blockage of the valve of Hasner at the nasal end of the nasolacrimal duct. Most of these obstructions resolve within the first 4 to 6 weeks of life. By the first year of life, approximately 90% of these will resolve.

Clinical Features

- Tearing in an infant
- Matting of the eyelashes
- Usually no conjunctival injection
- A dacryocystocoele may be present (a soft cystic lump located at the lower medial part of the eyelid), which is a non-infective collection of mucus in the lacrimal sac

Management

- Most cases are treated conservatively with Criggler's massage (downward pressure movements over the external skin region over the lacrimal sac). This is typically performed 10 times per day.
- If a dacryocystocoele is present, topical antibiotics can be used, along with Criggler's massage, or probing.
- When the NLDO fails to resolve with conservative measures, surgical intervention may be required.
- Probing of the nasolacrimal duct to perforate the membrane of the Valve of Hasner, re-establishing flow of tears. It is usually not done until the age of 6–12 months because spontaneous canalization may occur.
- Less commonly, other surgical procedures are required for persistent NLDO after probing. The probing can be repeated, and also combined with other procedures such as infracture of the nasal turbinates, intubation of the nasolacrimal duct, balloon dacryoplasty and even dacryocystorhinostomy for refractory cases of tearing due to NLDO.

Take home messages

- Acquired NLDO is surgically treated by endoscopic or external DCR.
- Congenital NLDO is a common condition that often spontaneously resolves with time.
- Conservative treatments such as massage and topical therapy is the mainstay of treatment.
- Surgical treatment is only indicated in a minority of cases, for refractory disease.

References

1. Bergin DJ. (1992) Lumps and bumps of the eyelids and their management. *J Dermatol Surg Oncol* **18**(12):1042–48.
2. Ellis E 3rd. (2012) Orbital trauma. *Oral Maxillofac Surg Clin North Am* **24**(4): 629–48.
3. Lim NC, Sundar G, Amrith S, *et al.* (2015) Thyroid eye disease: a Southeast Asian experience. *Br J Ophthalmol* **99**(4):512–18.
4. Sliverman N, Shinder R. (2017) What's new in eyelid tumors. *Asia-Pac J Ophthalmol* **6**:123–52.
5. Tailor TD, Gupta D, Dally RW, *et al.* (2013) Orbital neoplasms in adults: clinical, radiologic and pathologic review. *Radiographics* **33**(6): 1739-58.

Chapter 8

PAEDIATRIC OPHTHALMOLOGY AND STRABISMUS

8.1 Assessment of Vision in Children

Learning Objectives
- Understand visual milestones — from infancy to childhood.
- How to assess vision in an infant or child.
- How to recognize signs that may be a cause for concern.

Normal Visual Development in Children

Changes in Visual Acuity with Age

Born with an immature visual system, visual development begins within the first few weeks of life and continues to develop till the age of 8. Myelination of the optic nerves and maturation of the visual cortex occurs over the first 2 years of life. The fovea, the most visually sensitive part of the retina, reaches maturity at approximately 4 years of age.

Birth to 4 months of age

A *normal newborn* is usually born with poor vision due to immature visual centres in the brain and gradually develops the ability to focus on an object in front of him/her in the first few weeks of life. Development of good vision is dependent on well-focused images on the retina.

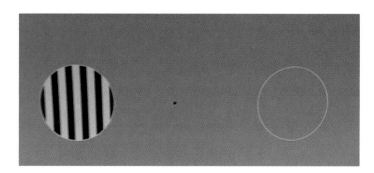

Fig. 8.1. Teller acuity cards — a type of forced preferential looking test for visual acuity

- At 1 month of age, a baby should be able to focus briefly on objects up to 1 metre away.
- By 2 months of age, infants should be able to track and follow moving objects, as their visual coordination and depth perception improves. However, it is not uncommon to notice a child's eyes to be deviated inwards or outwards up to 8 weeks of life, as their movements are still not well coordinated.
- By 3–4 months of age, distance vision continues to develop and an infant should be able to reach for objects around them and smile when they recognize a familiar face, e.g. a parent across the room.

Colour vision usually starts developing at birth and at one month of age, an infant can recognise intense colours and contrasting patterns (Fig. 8.1). By 4 months of age, they can differentiate and respond to the full range of shades and colours.

5–12 months of age

- During these months, the control of ocular movements and eye-body coordination skills continue to improve.
- Beyond 9 months of age, infants can start to judge distances fairly well and throw objects with precision.

1–2 years of age

During this period, a child's hand-eye coordination and depth perception should be well developed.

The visual system in children continues to be flexible throughout the first 8 years of life, thus treatment of amblyopia is best attempted before the age of 8. Any obstruction to focusing a clear image on the retina may lead to decreased vision and the development of amblyopia.

How to Assess Visual Acuity in a Young Infant

Children have low attention spans hence it is important to use objects that are attractive, high contrast, or colourful to get their attention.

It is difficult to assess vision in an infant but an estimation of gross visual function can be made. This is achieved by assessing an infant's ability to:

- **Fixate** on a visual object, **follow** it and maintain **steady** fixation. We usually record this as normal if an infant's gaze is **central, steady** and **maintained**.
- Blink/shy away from *bright light*.
- By 3–4 months, look for an infant's ability to **fixate on familiar faces**.
- Presence of *nystagmus* during this time usually indicates poorer vision.
- If there is objection to occlusion in either eye, it can be inferred that vision is fairly equal in both eyes (Fig. 8.2). However, if the baby objects only when one eye is covered, a difference in vision between the both eyes — with the better vision in the eye that objects to occlusion — must be suspected.
- A drum that induces physiological optokinetic response (*OKN drum,* Fig. 8.3) can be used to assess for normal vision. A horizontal OKN response is present by 3 months of age and a vertical OKN response should be expected by approximately 6 months of age.

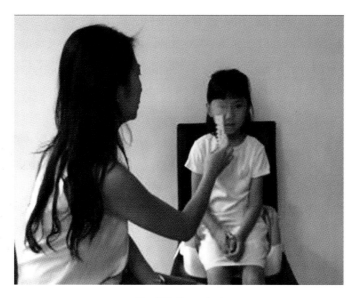

Fig. 8.2. Cover test.

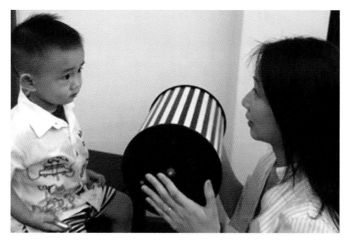

Fig. 8.3. Vertical optokinetic nystagmus testing using an OKN drum. If a vertical nystagmus can be elicited, vision is 6/120 or better.

Normal Visual Development in Children	Causes for Concern
• Birth → 6/300	• Wandering eyes/roving gaze
• 1 month → 6/200–6/90	• Presence of nystagmus
• 3 months 6/90–6/60	• Lack of response to familiar faces e.g. parents
• 6 months → FPL 6/60–6/36	• Staring straight at bright lights
• 9 months → FPL 6/36–6/24	• Oculodigital reflex
• 1 year → FPL 6/12	
• 2 years → FPL 6/12–6/9	
• 3 years → FPL 6/9–6/6	
• 4 years → FPL 6/6	

How to Assess Visual Acuity in a Child

Assessment of vision in a child requires age-appropriate methods of testing.

Type of Test	Age Tested	Name of Test	Example
Forced preferential looking (FPL) *Not suitable for children under the age of 6 months, uncooperative, has motor abnormalities e.g. nystagmus*	3 to 9 months	• Teller cards (grating) • Increasing	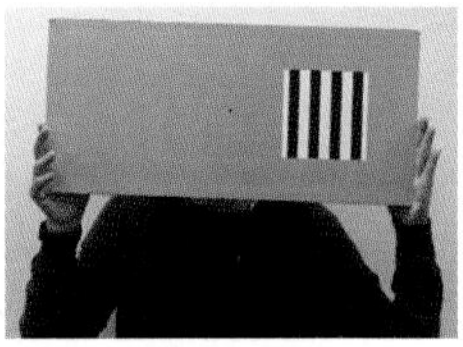 **Fig. 8.4**
	9 months to 2 years	• Cardiff cards (picture)	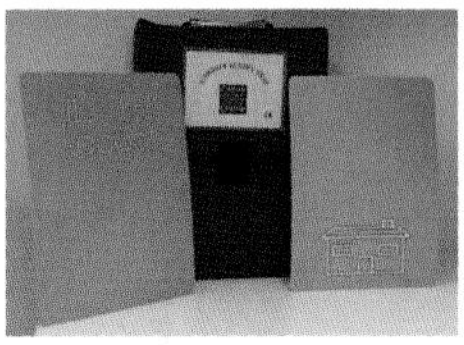 **Fig. 8.5**
Matching tests	2 to 4 years	• Kay picture cards	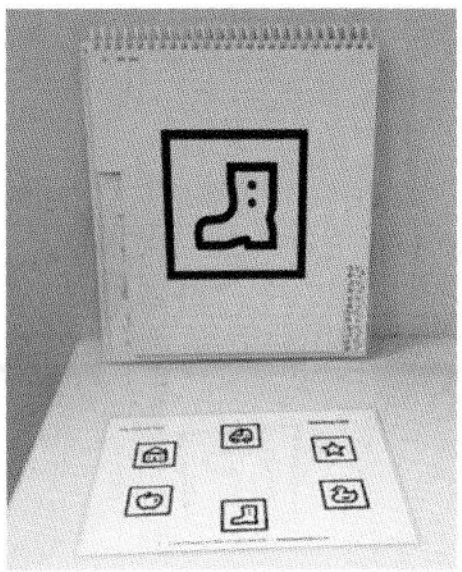 **Fig. 8.6**
	3 to 4 years	• Sheridan Gardiner (tests letters HOTUVXA)	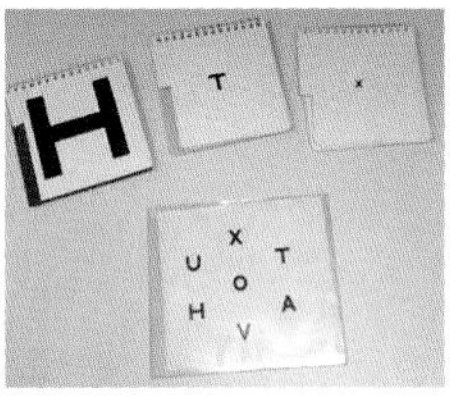 **Fig. 8.7**
Resolving ability of the eye	When child is able to recognize letters/ numbers	• Snellen chart • Using letters, numbers or tumbling E	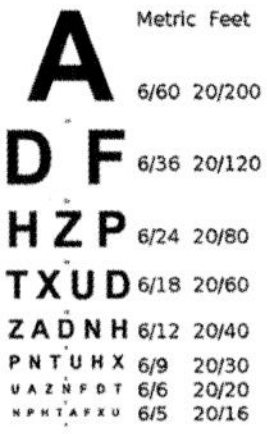 **Fig. 8.8**
		• Bailey Lovie (ETDRS, LogMAR)	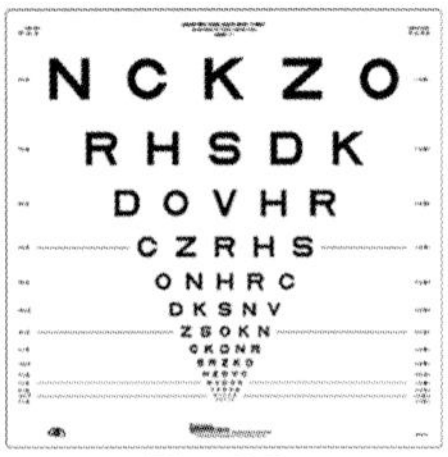 **Fig. 8.9**

Take home messages
- Normal newborns have poor vision and visual development occurs in the first few weeks of life.
- Assessment of vision in INFANTS
  - Fix + Follow, Gaze central, steady, maintained
  - Light → should blink/shy away from bright light
  - Faces → fixates on faces
  - Objection to Occlusion
  - Older infant → forced preferential looking
- Assessment of vision in CHILDREN
  - Forced Preferential Looking
  - Matching tests
  - Resolving ability of the eye → Snellen's chart, Bailey Lovie chart

8.2. Amblyopia

Learning Objectives
- Understand what is amblyopia.
- Note the causes of amblyopia.
- Understand the management of amblyopia.

Definition of Amblyopia/ "Lazy eye"

- Decreased vision in one or both eyes due to abnormal development of vision in infancy or childhood
- Visual acuity in either eye worse than 6/12 or if there is more than 2-line difference in visual acuity between the 2 eyes
- There may not be an obvious problem of the eye
- Vision loss occurs because nerve pathways between the brain and the eye are not properly stimulated
- The brain "learns" to see only blurry images with the amblyopic eye even when glasses are used
- As a result, the brain favours one eye, usually due to poor vision in the other eye

Causes of Amblyopia

- Strabismus or squint
- Vision deprivation, e.g.
  - Ptosis
    - i. Congenital ptosis
    - ii. Capillary hemangioma
  - Cataract

- Refractive error
  - Large refractive error or unequal amount of refractive error between both eyes
    - i. Large refractive error in both eyes → isoametropic amblyopia
    - ii. Unequal amount of refractive error between two eyes → anisometropic amblyopia
    - iii. High astigmatism causing amblyopia → meridional amblyopia

The end result of all forms of amblyopia is reduced vision in the affected eye(s)

Congenital ptosis
- A drooping eyelid that is present at birth (Fig. 8.10)
- The drooping eyelid can cover part or all of the pupil and interfere with vision, resulting in amblyopia
- Ptosis may also cause astigmatism, resulting in amblyopia as well
- Partial ptosis may be left alone; however, if ptosis causes astigmatism and occlusional/ deprivation amblyopia, spectacle correction is necessary as well as surgical treatment of congenital ptosis
  - Levator muscle resection
    - i. Shortening of the levator-aponeurosis complex through a lid-crease incision in those with moderate levator function
  - Frontalis suspension procedure
    - i. Augment the patient's lid elevation through brow elevation. The procedure is indicated when the levator function is poor

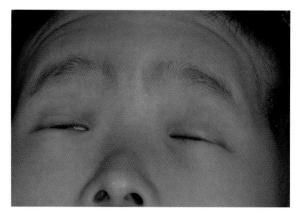

Fig. 8.10. Child with congenital ptosis and chin up head position.

Capillary/strawberry Hemangioma
- Benign tumour consisting of an abnormal overgrowth of tiny blood vessels
- May not be present at birth, but appear within the first 6 months of life
- Usually begin to decrease in size between 12 and 15 months of age. Most regress nearly completely by 5 or 6 years of age
- Eyelid hemangiomas may result in amblyopia by causing ptosis or astigmatism
- Orbital hemangiomas can compress the globe, eye muscles or optic nerve

- Treatment
  - No treatment may be necessary if there are no associated complications
  - Propranolol is taken orally but in some cases it can be applied topically if the hemangioma is very small and thin. Propranolol can affect heart rate and blood pressure, hence careful monitoring at the beginning of treatment is required
  - Steroids can stop the progression of hemangiomas by causing the blood vessels to shrink. Depending on the size and location of the hemangioma, steroids may be prescribed orally, injected directly into the hemangioma, or applied to the surface of the hemangioma. Steroid medications can have undesirable side effects including delayed physical growth, cataract, glaucoma and central retinal artery occlusion
  - Laser treatments can sometimes be used on superficial hemangiomas to prevent growth, diminish their size, or lighten their colour
  - Traditional surgery to remove hemangiomas around the eye is generally reserved for small, well-defined hemangiomas that are located under the skin surface

Assessment of Amblyopia

- Assessment of best corrected vision in a child requires age-appropriate methods of testing as outlined in Chapter 8.1
- Any refractive error should be tested using cycloplegic retinoscopy and corrected for and vision tested
- Ocular alignment should be assessed
- Full ophthalmologic assessment including dilated fundus examination should be carried out to rule out ocular pathologies that may contribute to decreased vision

Management of Amblyopia

- Early treatment is always best, before the age of 7–8
- If necessary, children with refractive errors (nearsightedness, farsightedness or astigmatism) can wear glasses
- Children with cataracts, squints or other "amblyogenic" conditions are usually treated promptly
- SOME improvement in vision can be attained with amblyopia therapy initiated in younger teenagers (through age 14 years)
- Patching of the better seeing eye to allow the weak eye to get stronger
- "Penalize" or blur the stronger (good) eye with atropine eye drops temporally

---

Take home messages
- Amblyopia is decreased vision in one or both eyes due to abnormal development of vision.
- Causes include strabismus, vision deprivation or refractive errors.
- Management
  - Patching of the better seeing eye to allow the weak eye to get stronger.
  - "Penalize" or blur the stronger (good) eye with atropine eye drops.

8.3 Strabismus

Learning Objectives
• How to assess strabismus.
• Causes and management of eso- and exo- deviations.
• Principles of strabismus management.

Assessment of Strabismus

Strabismus

• Misalignment of the eyes which may be
  ▪ Horizontal
  ▪ Vertical
  ▪ Torsional
• Nomenclature (Fig. 8.11)
  ▪ Orthophoria (straight)
  ▪ Esotropia (manifest convergent strabismus; seen on cover test)
  ▪ Esophoria (latent convergent strabismus; seen only on alternate cover test)
  ▪ Exotropia (manifest divergent strabismus; seen on cover test)
  ▪ Exophoria (latent divergent strabismus; seen only on alternate cover test)
  ▪ Intermittent Exotropia (manifest divergent strabismus which occurs at times; seen on cover test)
  ▪ Right Hypertropia (named after the higher eye; seen on cover test)

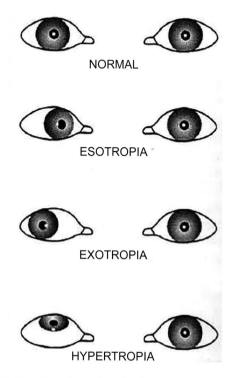

Fig. 8.11. Hirschberg test using a bright co-axial light source.

- Clinical presentation
  - Abnormal head posture
  - Head tilt
  - Face turn
  - Facial asymmetry
- Binocular red reflex (Bruckner)
  - A bright coaxial light source, such as a direct ophthalmoscope, is used. Both eyes of the patient are simultaneously illuminated from approximately one meter distance. When strabismus is present, the fixing eye has a darker reflex than the deviated eye
- Hirschberg test (corneal light reflex)
  - A bright coaxial light source, such as a direct ophthalmoscope, is used. The position of the corneal light reflex is evaluated (Fig. 8.11 and Fig. 8.12)
  - Normal: slight symmetrical nasal displacement of 5 degrees

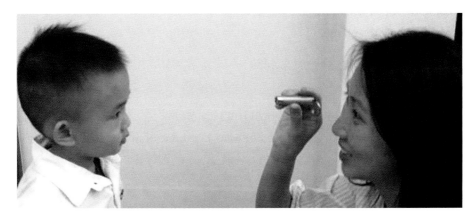

Fig. 8.12. Hirschberg test — checking for the corneal light reflex using a bright pentorch.

- Cover test/Uncover test
  - Detect tropia
  - Patient to fixate on an object
  - Cover normal eye (1–2 sec) and observe the abnormal eye for shift to midline
- Alternate cover test
  - Dissociate binocular fusion to determine full deviation (tropia and phoria)
  - Alternately occlude each eye, observe for refixation shift of uncovered eye to midline

Esodeviation (Inturn of the Eyes)

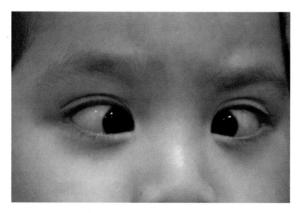

Fig. 8.13. Bilateral esotropia.

Infantile Esotropia (Fig. 8.13)

- Onset first 6 months of age
- Large angle
- Amblyopia in 50%
- Early surgery usually required
- Poor prognosis for high grade stereopsis/3D vision
- Usually require second surgery for other associated motor anomalies

Accomodative Esotropia

- Far-sighted (Fig. 8.14A)
- Increase focusing effort to see clearly
- Acquired between 3–6 months and 5 years of age
- Hypermetropic glasses
  - Straight after hypermetropic glasses
    (Fully accomodative esotropia, Fig. 8.14B)
    - i. Good prognosis for stereoacuity and binocular fusion
  - Residual ET after full hypermetropic glasses
    (Partially accomodative esotropia, Fig. 8.14C)
    - – Surgery needed

Exodeviation

- Intermittent exodeviation common (Fig. 8.14E)
- Between age 2–8
- Occurs when child tired/day dreaming
- Vague eye discomfort, photophobia, squinting
- Good stereopsis and binocular fusion when eyes aligned (Fig. 8.14D)
- Requires surgery if poorly controlled

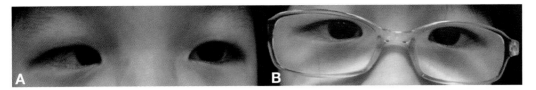

Fig. 8.14A & B. In this child with accommodative right esotropia, the right esotropia resolves with fitting the child with a pair of hyperopic glasses to relax the accommodation.

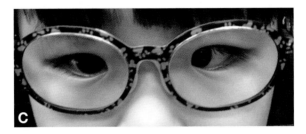

Fig. 8.14C. Residual left esotropia is seen in the child with partially accommodative esotropia

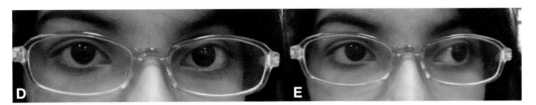

Fig. 8.14D & E. Intermittent exotropia.

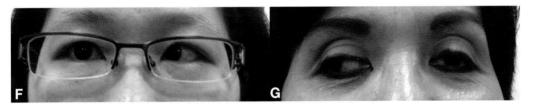

Fig. 8.14F & G. Esodeviations and exodeviations may result from poor vision in the deviating eye.

Sensory Deviation

- Loss of vision causes an eye to drift
- Visual loss < 2 years of age usually leads to esotropia (Fig. 8.14F)
- Visual loss > 2 years of age usually leads to exotropia (Fig. 8.14G)

Complications of Strabismus

- Acquired: diplopia/ double vision
- Before age 6: cortical suppression of image from deviated eye
  - Strabismic amblyopia
  - Loss of binocular fusion and stereopsis

- Dangerous strabismus
  - Acquired strabismus
  - Associated with diplopia
  - Limited eye movements
  - Ptosis or other neurological signs
  - Poor vision
  - Abnormal red reflex

Principles of Strabismus Management

- Prescribe glasses if necessary
- Treat lazy eye: patching
- Orthoptic exercises
- Prisms for diplopia
- Surgery
  - Aims:
    - i. Achieve binocular single vision
    - ii. Eliminate head posture
    - iii. Cosmesis
  - Slacken muscle (e.g. recession)
  - Tighten muscle (e.g. resection, plication)
  - Reduce length of moment arm (Faden)
  - Change the vector of muscle force by moving the muscle's insertion site (transposition)

Take home messages
- Strabismus can be detected using Hirschberg test as well as cover tests.
- Acquired strabismus or those associated with neurological signs and poor vision must be investigated urgently.
- Management of strabismus should start with glasses and patching first if necessary, orthoptics exercises and prisms for diplopia.
- Surgery for strabismus can be considered for diplopia, abnormal head posture, worsening angles of deviation of strabismus or decreasing stereopsis, or cosmetically unacceptable strabismus.

8.4 Leukocoria

Learning Objectives
- Understand important causes of leukocoria.
- Understand presentation and assessment of retinoblastoma.
- Understand presentation and assessment of congenital cataracts.

Approach to Leukocoria

Presence of a "white pupil," name given to the clinical finding of a white pupillary reflex (Fig. 8.15), when the path of light is obstructed in the eye.

Causes of Leucokoria

- Lens
  - Cataract
- Vitreous
  - Persistent foetal vasculature
- Retina
  - Retinoblastoma
  - Non accidental Injury
  - Coats' disease
  - Retinopathy of prematurity
  - Optic disc abnormalities
  - Congenital infections (toxoplasmosis, toxocara)

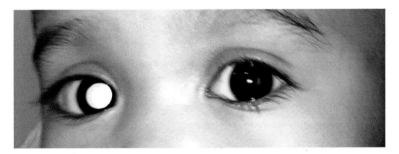

Fig. 8.15. Right eye leukocoria.

Assessment of Leukocoria

- All children with newly discovered leukocoria should urgently be referred to an ophthalmologist
- History
  - Prenatal exposures (toxins, infection, medications) and complications
  - Birth history
  - Postnatal course (infection, oxygen exposure, medications)
  - Medical history, growth pattern, development, and review of systems

- Recent exposures (puppies, kittens, medications)
- Family history (particularly for retinoblastoma or other eye diseases, eye loss, osteogenic sarcoma, and foetal loss or miscarriage)
- Physical examination including dysmorphic features; growth parameters; signs of coagulopathy, trauma, or neurocutaneous disorders; and organomegaly.
  - Age-appropriate vision assessment and external examination (See Chapter 8.1)
  - Anterior segment and dilated fundoscopic examination
- Radiologic testing
  - Ophthalmic ultrasonography is routinely used to determine the presence or absence of an intraocular mass with associated intralesional calcium, which is indicative of retinoblastoma

Retinoblastoma

Epidemiology
- Most common intraocular malignancy (Fig. 8.16) in children
- Incidence of one in 15–20,000 live births
- Average age of presentation — 18 months
  - Bilateral — 13 months
  - Unilateral — 24 months
  - Family history — 11 months

Genetics
- 40% hereditary
- Autosomal dominant germline mutation of RB1 gene (tumour suppressor gene) on 13q14
- Two active copies of the retinoblastoma gene are normally carried in human cells. Both copies must be mutated to lead to the development of retinoblastoma
- The initial mutation inactivates one copy of the gene. This mutation may occur in somatic or germline cells. The second mutation occurs in somatic cells

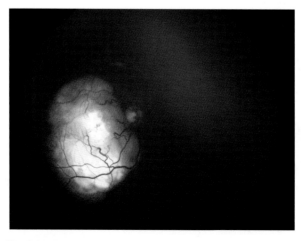

Fig. 8.16. Retinoblastoma of the right eye involving the macula.

Presentation

- Leukocoria in 50%
- Strabismus
- Change in eye appearance (heterochromia or red, painful, or watery eyes)
- Reduced visual acuity

Assessment

- MRI (Fig. 8.17)
  - Involvement of optic nerve
  - Pineal gland (PNET)
  - Other eye
- Evaluate cerebrospinal fluid (CSF) and bone marrow when the child is at risk for metastatic disease
- Staging examination under anaesthesia (EUA)
  - Retcam
  - Ophthalmic ultrasonography (B scan; Fig. 8.18)
  - Fundus fluorescein angiogram
- Genetic testing/counselling

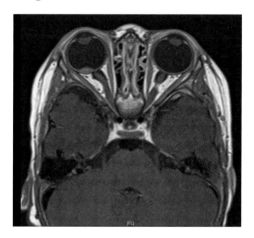

Fig. 8.17. MRI showing retinoblastoma of the right eye not involving the optic nerve.

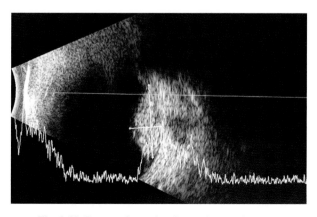

Fig. 8.18. B scan of eye showing an intraocular mass.

Management

- Preservation of life before globe, before vision
- Multimodality multidisciplinary management
  - Enucleation
  - Chemo reduction (systemic, local, intra-arterial)
  - Local (laser photocoagulation, cryotherapy)
  - Genetic testing

Congenital Cataracts (Fig. 8.19)

Aetiology

- Systemic
  - Genetic (Down syndrome, trisomy 13/15)
  - Metabolic (Lowe syndrome, galactosemia)
  - Infections (Rubella, CMV, HSV, Toxoplasmosis)
- Ocular
- Toxic
  - Steroids
  - Radiation

Assessment

- VA-fixates on light? Any objection to occlusion?
- Red reflex
- Ophthalmoscopy through undilated pupil
  - Central opacity or surrounding cortical distortion > 3 mm is visually significant
- Laboratory Tests
  - TORCH (toxoplasma, rubella, CMV, herpes) and varicella titers
  - VDRL (for syphilis)
  - Serum calcium, phosphorus, glucose and ferritin
  - Urine for reducing substance, galactose 1-phosphate uridyltransferase, galactokinase, amino acids

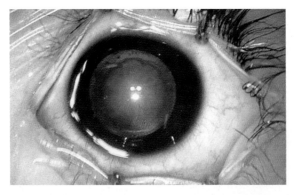

Fig. 8.19. Intraoperative photograph showing the presence of a lamellar cataract in a young infant.

Management

- Surgery
  - Visually significant cataract
  - Between 4–6 weeks of age
  - If bilateral, second eye 1 week after the first
- Post-op
  - Refractive correction
    - i. Glasses (bilateral)
    - ii. Contact lens
  - Aggressive amblyopia treatment if unilateral

Non Accidental Injury/Shaken Baby Syndrome

- Suspect when
  - Injury is unexplained
  - Severity of the injury incompatible with history
  - History keeps changing
  - Injury is inconsistent with the developmental age
  - Delay in seeking medical care following an injury
  - Suspected abuse needs to be thoroughly investigated with the assistance of child protection services

Associated features

- Bruising
- Burns
- Fractures
- Abusive head trauma
  - Intracranial haemorrhage
  - Diffuse retinal haemorrhage (Fig. 8.20)
    - i. Often multilayered
    - ii. Occur in 60–85 % of non-accidental head injuries
    - iii. Uncommon in accidental head trauma

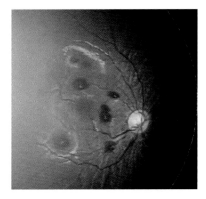

Fig. 8.20. Fundus photograph of the right eye in a child who sustained multiple retinal hemorrhages after a non-accidental injury.

- Diffuse brain injury.
  i. Signs and symptoms may be non-specific, such as vomiting, poor feeding, irritability or lethargy
- May have no external signs of injury

Retinopathy of Prematurity (ROP)

- Retinal vascularisation on the internal retinal surface begins at the optic nerve at 16 weeks gestation and proceeds anteriorly
  - Reaches nasal retina by 36 weeks
  - Reaches temporal retina by 40 weeks
- Screening
  - All premature babies < 1500g, < 32 weeks gestation age
  - 1st check 4-6 weeks after birth; after 31 weeks gestation age
- Risk Factors
  - Small for gestational age
  - Low birth weight
  - Longer duration of artificial ventilation
  - Multiple births
  - Respiratory distress
  - Congenital heart disease
  - Post natal anaemia
  - Intracranial haemorrhage
  - Apnoea
  - Exchange transfusion
  - Perinatal hypoxia
  - Sepsis
  - Intrauterine growth retardation
- Zones and extent (Fig. 8.21)
  - Zone I is a circle, the radius of which extends from the centre of the optic disc to twice the distance from the center of the optic disc to the centre of the macula
  - Zone II extends centrifugally from the edge of zone I to the nasal ora serrata
  - Zone III is the residual temporal crescent of retina anterior to zone II
  - Stage 1: Demarcation Line
    i. Line that separates the avascular retina anteriorly from the vascularized retina posteriorly
  - Stage 2: Ridge
    i. The ridge arises from the demarcation line and has height and width
  - Stage 3: Extraretinal fibrovascular proliferation
    i. Neovascularisation extends from the ridge into the vitreous.
  - Stage 4: Partial retinal detachment (Fig. 8.22)
  - Stage 5: Total retinal detachment

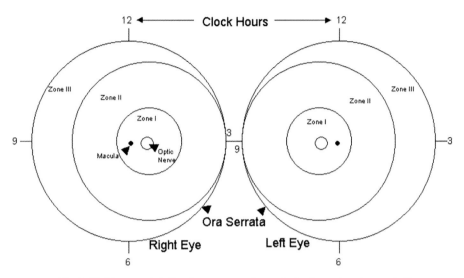

Fig. 8.21. Diagram detailing the zones and extent of retinopathy of prematurity.

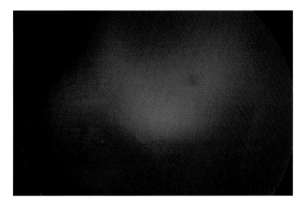

Fig. 8.22. Stage 4 retinopathy of prematurity showing a partial retinal detachment.

- Treatment
  - Laser therapy
  - Intravitreal anti-VEGF (vascular endothelial growth factor)

Take home messages
- Prompt diagnosis and treatment are important in leukocoria.
- All children with newly discovered leukocoria should urgently be referred to an ophthalmologist.
- The most important cause of leukocoria is retinoblastoma.

8.5 Tearing and Discharge in an Infant / Young Child

Learning Objectives
• Understand the common and sight threatening causes of tearing in an infant or young child.
• How to assess tearing in an infant or young child.

Approach to Tearing in an Infant/Young Child

Nasolacrimal duct obstruction (NLDO) is the most common cause of persistent tearing in an infant/ young child, and can lead to infection and ocular discharge. Other causes range from mild, self-limiting conditions (e.g. allergic conjunctivitis) to severe sight-threatening ocular emergencies (e.g. ophthalmia neonatorum).

Causes of Tearing in an Infant/Young Child

Aetiology of tearing in a child can be congenital or acquired, and occur secondary to either *hypersecretion* of the tear glands or *obstruction* of the tear drainage system (Fig. 8.23).

The causes of tearing can also be classified as follows:

Sight threatening causes	Congenital glaucoma Ophthalmia neonatorum
Common causes	NLDO Conjunctivitis, frequently allergic
Others	Corneal or conjunctival foreign body/abrasion Eyelid abnormalities Epiblepharon causing lash-corneal touch Trichiasis / districhiasis Entropion Blepharitis

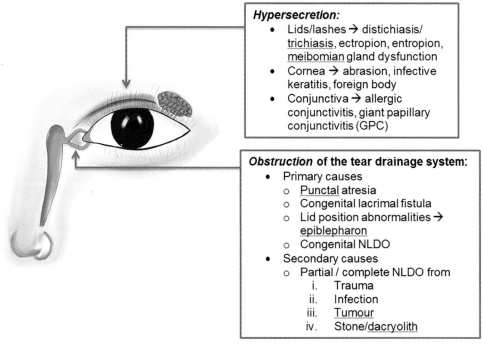

Hypersecretion:
• Lids/lashes → distichiasis/ trichiasis, ectropion, entropion, meibomian gland dysfunction
• Cornea → abrasion, infective keratitis, foreign body
• Conjunctiva → allergic conjunctivitis, giant papillary conjunctivitis (GPC)

Obstruction of the tear drainage system:
• Primary causes
   o Punctal atresia
   o Congenital lacrimal fistula
   o Lid position abnormalities → epiblepharon
   o Congenital NLDO
• Secondary causes
   o Partial / complete NLDO from
      i. Trauma
      ii. Infection
      iii. Tumour
      iv. Stone/dacryolith

Fig. 8.23. Causes of tearing in an infant or young child.

Assessment of Tearing in an Infant/Young Child

History

- Onset (acute / gradual), progression
- Type of discharge: watery, purulent
- Past medical history: previous sinus surgery/disease, trauma, dacryocystitis
- Previous surgery/ radiation

Examination

Examine the patient under the slit lamp, looking for:
- Eyelids: entropion, ectropion, distichiasis, trichiasis, lid laxity
- Punctum: well apposed to tear lake/ globe, atresia
- Tear film — oily, high or low
- Cornea / Conjunctiva — ulcers, infiltrates, punctate epithelial erosions, abrasions, giant papillary conjunctivitis
- Intraocular pressure (IOP) — suggestive of glaucoma

Fluorescein tests

- Level of tear film
- Fluorescein dye disappearance test (FDDT)
  - Instill 2% fluorescein eyedrop
  - After 5 minutes, check for dye to disappear
  - Delay in disappearance → problem lies in tear drainage system
- Jones I test
  - Check for fluorescein in the nose with cotton swabstick
  - Lack of fluorescein in nose would suggest a partial/complete NLDO

Other investigations

- Nasal endoscopy → look for dye under inferior turbinate within inferior meatus (may be difficult in young children)
- Syringing and probing
  - Done under general anaesthesia in young children
  - Check for presence of punctal atresia / stenosis
  - Soft / hard stop
    - i. Soft stop → suggestive of proximal NLDO
    - ii. Hard stop → suggestive of distal NLDO
  - Presence of reflux

Congenital Nasolacrimal Duct Obstruction

Please refer to chapter in "Oculoplastics" (Chapter 7.3)

Congenital Glaucoma

Please refer to chapter in Glaucoma (Chapter 4.2)

Ophthalmia Neonatorum

Causes

- Infections:
  - Bacterial
    - i. Most common → *Neisseria gonorrhoea, Chlamydia trachomatis*
    - ii. Others → *Staphylococcus aureus, Streptococcus penumoniae, Streptococcus viridans, Staphylococcus epidermidis, Hemophilus influenzae,* enterococcus, *Escherichia coli, Klebsiella, Serratia, Pseudomonas aeruginosa*
  - Viral
    - i. Herpes simplex virus (1–2 weeks after birth, vesicles on face, herpetic dendritic keratitis)
- Chemical:
  - Usually presents within first 24 hours
  - Types →
    - i. Silver nitrate
    - ii. Erythromycin, tetracycline
  - Self limiting, resolves within 1–2 days
- Trauma

Time frame of signs/ symptoms following the birth of a child can play an important role in determining the most likely aetiology in ophthalmia neonatorum			
Chemical conjunctivitis	*Neisseria gonorrhoea*	*Chlamydia trachomatis*	Herpes simplex virus (HSV)
Within 24 hours after birth	3–5 days after birth	5–14 days after birth	1–2 weeks after birth

Assessment

- Things to ask for in history
  - Symptoms/Signs, e.g. eye redness, discharge
  - Duration, laterality, progression
  - Visual behaviour
  - Maternal infections, e.g. vaginal discharge
  - Mode of delivery — ophthalmia neonatorum commonly acquired through passage of baby through birth canal
  - Any birth complications
- Things to look out for in examination
  - Take conjunctival swabs before performing eye lavage
  - Examine the eye for
    - Conjunctival redness, chemosis
    - Corneal epithelial defect, infiltrate, perforation
    - Purulent discharge
    - Anterior segment for hypopyon
    - Dilated fundal examination

- Check the child systemically
  - Signs of meningitis — fever / sepsis / neck stiffness
- Investigate for the cause
  - Send the conjunctival swabs for microbiological diagnosis
    - Gram stain
    - Cultures and sensitivities
    - *Chlamydia* immunofluorescence / polymerase chain reaction (PCR)
    - *Neisseria gonorrhoea* PCR
  - Blood cultures if child is septic
  - Conjunctival swabs for mother if she has symptoms suggestive of pelvic inflammatory disease

Management

- Co-manage this patient with a paediatrician to rule out systemic involvement → refer to Paediatrics Infectious Disease
- Counsel the mother about the need to start topical broad spectrum antibiotics, e.g. Tobramycin eyedrops
- Teach the mother to toilet eye hourly with saline lavage
- Close follow up → review the child daily until cultures are available
  - Tailor treatment according to culture results / sensitivity
- Treat the child and parents
  - Child →
    - i. Chlamydia : Oral erythromycin 50 mg / kg / day in divided doses Q6H x 2 weeks
    - ii. Gonorrhea : IV / IM ceftriaxone 50 mg / kg / day in divided or single dose x 7 days
    - iii. Herpetic : Oral acyclovir 30 mg / kg / day in 3 divided doses x 2 weeks
      - Admit
      - Topical acyclovir as well
  - Adult →
    - i. Chlamydia
      - Oral azithromycin 1 g x (1 dose) or
      - Oral doxycycline 100 mg BD x (7 days)
    - ii. Gonococcal
      - IM ceftriaxone 250 mg x (1 dose) + oral azithromycin 1 g (1 dose) or
      - Oral doxycycline 100 mg BD x (7 days)

Systemic Manifestations

Ophthalmia neonatorum may be associated with systemic manifestations if due to bacterial cause.

- Gonorrhoea
  - Meningitis
  - Arthritis
  - Septicaemia
  - Stomatitis, rhinitis

- Chlamydia
  - Pneumonitis
  - Otitis media
  - Pharyngeal
  - Rectal colonisation

Orbital Cellulitis in Children

Please refer to chapter on "Oculoplastics" (Chapter 7.2)

> **Take home messages**
> - Glaucoma in an infant/ young child can present with tearing and can lead to blindness if left untreated.
> - The *most common cause* of excessive tearing in an infant is nasolacrimal duct obstruction.
> - *Important sight threatening causes* of tearing in a young child/infant are congenital glaucoma, orbital cellulitis and ophthalmia neonatorum.

8.6 Refractive Error

> **Learning Objectives**
> - Understand how to prescribe refractive correction for children.
> - Know the definitions of emmetropia, ametropia, hyperopia, myopia and astigmatism.
> - Know how to read a refraction prescription.

Prescribing for Children

- In adults, the correction of refractive errors has 1 measurable endpoint: the best corrected visual acuity
- In children, however, correction of refractive errors has 2 goals:
  - Provide a focused image on the retina
  - Achieve optimal balance between accommodation and convergence
- Techniques of refraction in children:
  - Subjective refraction
    i. Can be performed in older children
    ii. Difficult in infants and young children due to their inability to cooperate with subjective refraction techniques
  - Objective refraction
    i. Optimal technique of refraction in infants and small children
    ii. Requires paralysis of accommodation with complete cycloplegia

Definition of Emmetropia, Ametropia, Hyperopia, Myopia and Astigmatism

Emmetropia (Fig. 8.24)

- Refractive state in which parallel rays of light from a distant object are brought to focus on the retina in the non-accommodating eye

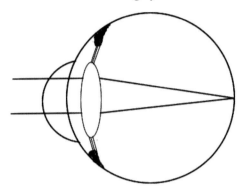

Fig. 8.24. Emmetropia with accommodation relaxed.

Ametropia

- Absence of emmetropia
- Can be classified as axial or refractive
  - i. Axial ametropia — the eyeball is either unusually long (axial myopia) or short (axial hyperopia)
  - ii. Refractive ametropia — the eyeball is statistically normal but the refractive power of the eye (cornea and/or lens) is abnormal, being either excessive (refractive myopia) or deficient (refractive hyperopia)

Hyperopia (Fig. 8.25)

- Can be axial or refractive
- Eye possesses insufficient optical power for its axial length, hence in the non-accommodating eye, the light rays from an object at infinity attempts to focus light behind the retina
- Usually expressed with a "plus" sign in diopters (D)

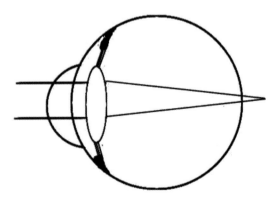

Fig. 8.25. Hyperopia with accommodation relaxed.

Myopia (Fig. 8.26)

- Can be axial or refractive
- Eye possesses too much optical power for its axial length hence, in the non-accommodating eye, the light rays from an object at infinity converge and focus in front of the retina
- Usually expressed with a "minus" sign in diopters (D)

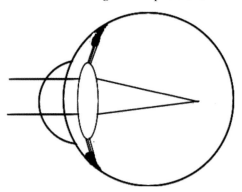

Fig. 8.26. Myopia with accommodation relaxed.

Astigmatism

- Optical condition of the eye in which light rays from an object do not focus to a single point because of variations in the curvature of the cornea or lens at different meridians, resulting in a set of 2 focal lines
- Usually expressed with a "minus" sign in diopters (D) with an axis ranging from 0 to 180 degrees (orientation of meridian of greatest curvature)

How to Read a Refraction Prescription

- Looking at a prescription for refraction, numbers are listed under headings of **Right or Left eye, or OD and OS** (Latin abbreviations)
  - OD —oculus dextrus— means right eye
  - OS —oculus sinister— means left eye
  - Occasionally a notation for OU may be seen, which means involving both eyes
- **Spherical (SPH) component**
  - Plus sign — signifies hyperopia
  - Minus sign — signifies myopia
  - Numbers represent diopters, the unit used to measure the refractive correction or focusing power that the eye requires
    i. Diopter: often abbreviated as "D"
- **Cylinder (CYL) component**
  - A measure of the amount of astigmatism one has
  - Axis: ranges from 0 to 180 degrees
    i. Reveals the orientation of the astigmatism to meridian of greatest curvature (usually referring to the cornea)

- **Near Add component**
  - Needed when accommodative amplitude is insufficient for the patient to read or carry out near-vision tasks
  - Can also be given to children who have a high accommodative convergence to accommodation ratio (AC:A ratio)
  - Usually expressed with "plus" sign as convex lenses are needed for correction

Example of a refraction prescription:

Cylinder:
Presence of 1 diopter
of cylinder with axis of
greatest curvature at
180 degrees

Near Add:
This patient requires
2.50 diopters of convex
lenses to achieve a
near vision of N5

Right Eye (OD)					
Sph (D)	Cyl (D)	Axis (degrees)	VA (visual acuity)	Near Add (D)	VA (visual acuity)
+3.00	-1.00	180	6/6	+2.50	N5

Sphere:
Signifies this patient
requires 3 diopters to
correct the hyperopia

Best corrected visual
acuity that patient can
see with this refractive
corrrection

Take home messages
- Refraction in children may be achieved by either subjective or objective refraction techniques.
- Reading a refraction prescription:
  - Has both Spherical and Cylindrical component
  - Plus sign – signifies Hyperopia
  - Minus sign – signifies Myopia
  - Numbers represent diopters, the unit used to measure the refractive correction or focusing power that the eye requires.
    i. Diopter – often abbreviated as "D".

References

1. American Academy of Ophthalmology (AAO). 2016–2017 Edition. *Paediatric Ophthalmology and Strabismus*, and *Orbit, Eyelids and Lacrimal system* chapters.

2. American Academy of Ophthalmology (AAO). 2016–2017 Edition. Clinical Optics & Paediatric Ophthalmology and Strabismus chapters.

3. American Optometric Association. www.aoa.org

4. Approach to the child with persistent tearing. www.uptodate.com

5. Normal Vision Development in Babies and Children. www.aao.org

6. *Practical Ophthalmology — A manual for Beginning Residents* (AAO); Fourth Edition. Fred M. Wilson, *et al.*

7. *The Ophthalmology Examinations Review*, 2nd ed. TY Wong

Chapter 9

NEURO-OPHTHALMOLOGY

Neuro-ophthalmology is a challenging and fascinating branch of ophthalmology. The clinical cases are diverse in presentation. Good knowledge of neuro-anatomy (Chapter 1), ophthalmology, neurology, neurosurgery, general medicine and radiology is required to determine the site and elucidate the cause of the disease.

This chapter aims to provide an overview of and approach to the important Neuro-ophthalmic conditions that non-ophthalmologists may encounter.

9.1 Optic Neuropathy

Learning Objectives
- To be able to recognise that optic neuropathy is a possible cause of visual loss.
- To be able to clinically determine normal, swollen and pale optic discs(s), and to list differentials for each

Evaluation of a Patient with Suspected Optic Neuropathy

The term "optic neuropathy" refers to dysfunction of the optic nerve(s), without specifically describing the cause (or aetiology). A large number of conditions may cause optic neuropathy.

Optic neuropathy can present in a variety of ways. Patients may report loss of vision, darkening of vision, change in colour saturation or something that "does not feel right." Patients with optic neuropathies are typically found to have loss of visual acuity, visual field defects, dyschromatopsia and a relative afferent pupillary defect in varying combination.

When evaluating patients with possible optic neuropathy, it is crucial to take a thorough history and perform a complete ophthalmic and neurological examination. In addition, investigations are usually needed to aid the clinician with diagnosis, and subsequent follow up.

History
- Visual loss — onset, progression, severity
- Pain — headache, pain on eye movement
- History of trauma
- Past medical history—vascular risk factors, malignancy, family history
- Dietary and medication history, including supplements and traditional medicines
- Social history — smoking, alcohol consumption, illicit drugs

Examination

- Vital signs of optic nerve function:
  - Visual acuity
  - Pupillary function (Is there a *RAPD?)
  - Colour vision
  - Visual fields

*Note that a RAPD is practically always present when there is a unilateral optic neuropathy unless there is equally severe loss of vision from retina or macular disease in the fellow eye.

- Anterior and posterior segment examination: particularly of the optic disc
- Intraocular pressure
- Neurological examination (particularly the cranial nerves): is this an isolated optic neuropathy or are other parts of the nervous system involved?

Investigations

- Perimetry — Humphrey visual fields (static perimetry) or Goldman visual fields (kinetic perimetry)
- Optical coherence tomography (OCT) of the disc and macula
- Neuroimaging — magnetic resonance imaging (MRI) / computed tomography (CT), with or without accompanying vascular studies
- Imaging of the fundus / optic disc is useful for documentation and follows up

The appearance of the optic disc, though important, does not usually give a direct indication of the underlying pathology. Optic neuropathies can present with a normal looking disc (Fig. 9.1), a swollen disc, a pale disc, or a cupped disc (Fig. 9.2). Disc swelling may indicate inflammation, ischaemia or raised intracranial pressure. A pale disc simply indicates a past or chronic, on-going insult to the optic nerve. Optic disc cupping is typically seen in glaucoma, but may also be the result of other diseases. An outline of the causes of the swollen or pale disc is given in Table 9.1.

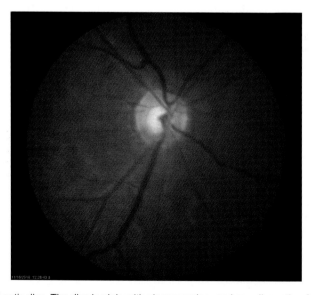

Fig. 9.1. A normal optic disc. The disc is pink, with clear margins, and cup disc ratio of approximately 0.4.

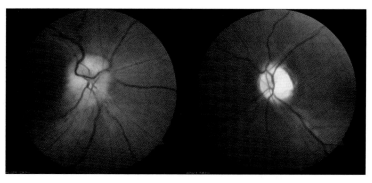

Patient 1 — right swollen disc and left pale disc from sequential ischaemic optic neuropathies.

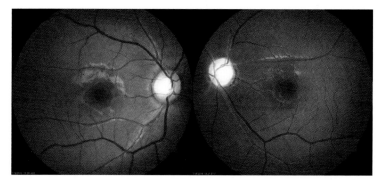

Patient 2 — bilateral slightly cupped discs and left pale disc from an optic disc glioma

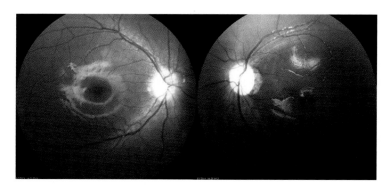

Patient 3 — bilateral pale discs from inflammatory optic neuropathy.

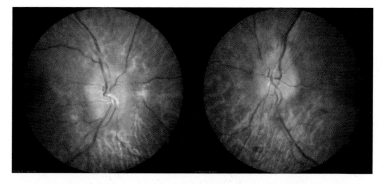

Patient 4 — bilateral swollen discs from raised intracranial pressure.

Fig. 9.2. Various presentations of optic neuropathies.

Table 9.1. Causes of Swollen and Pale Optic Discs

Swollen Disc(s)		Pale Disc(s)	
Unilateral	**Bilateral**	**Unilateral**	**Bilateral**
• Ischaemic • Inflammatory* • Compressive* • Infiltrative* • Radiation* • Others: CRVO	• Malignant Hypertension# • Raised intracranial pressure (ICP)# ▪ Identifiable intracranial pathology ▪ Idiopathic • Venous Sinus Thrombosis #	• Compressive • Traumatic • Ischaemic∞ • Inflammatory∞ • Infiltrative∞ • Radiation • Toxic / nutritional	• Hereditary • Toxic / nutritional • Compressive • Radiation
* May occasionally be bilateral	# May also cause unilateral disc swelling	∞Sequential past insult may result in bilateral pale discs	

Clinical Presentation of Optic Neuropathies

Optic Disc Swelling

A swollen disc is due to nerve oedema from obstruction of axoplasmic flow; which may result from ischaemia, inflammation, compression, metabolic, or toxic disorders. Signs of disc swelling include obscuration of vessels crossing the optic disc, blurring of disc margins, hyperaemia, haemorrhages and exudates.

Patient presentation is dependent on the cause of optic disc swelling. Disc swelling from ischaemic or inflammatory optic neuropathies (optic neuritis) usually presents with acute visual loss. Disc swelling from compressive or infiltrative optic neuropathies may present with painless, progressive visual loss. Patients with papilloedema (disc swelling caused by raised intracranial pressure (ICP)) often present with transient visual obscuration or symptoms of raised ICP such as headache and vomiting. The blood pressure is severely elevated in patients with malignant hypertension.

Not all disc swelling represents an isolated optic neuropathy. A dilated fundus examination is necessary in all patients to determine if there is other intraocular pathology. Figure 9.3 illustrates three patients who had optic disc swelling secondary to other intraocular diseases.

The optic disc may sometimes appear on fundoscopic examination to be swollen even though there is no actual thickening of the retinal nerve fibre layer. Such pseudo disc swelling

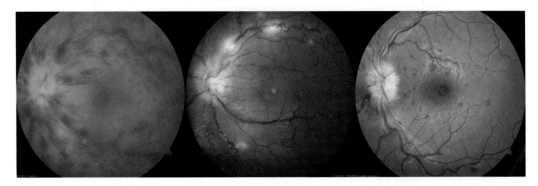

Fig. 9.3. From *left* to *right*: central retinal vein occlusion, retinal vasculitis and lymphoproliferative disorder.

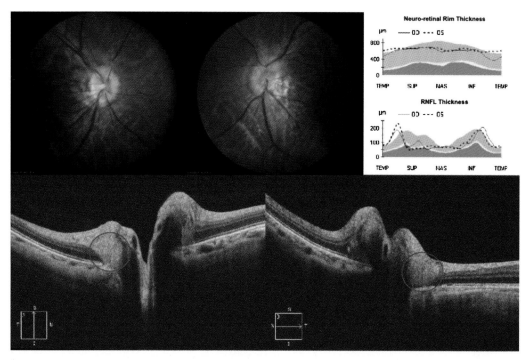

Fig. 9.4. Both optic disc look swollen in the photos. However, the retinal nerve fibre layer (RNFL) is not elevated, and there are drusen (red circles) seen on the OCT.

may be the result of a congenitally small, crowded disc or optic disc drusen. Figure 9.4 illustrates a patient who had a normal MRI brain, cerebrospinal fluid (CSF) opening pressure and composition, and was found to have optic disc drusen on OCT of the discs (red circles).

Before attributing the appearance of a swollen optic disc to pseudo-swelling, it is necessary to ensure that there are no signs and symptoms of visual loss or raised intracranial pressure, and preferably obtain imaging of the retinal nerve fibre layer to monitor for progression.

Optic Disc Pallor

A pale disc represents previous optic nerve injury. It is generally held that disc pallor sets in 6 weeks or more after insult to the optic nerve.

The management of patients with optic disc pallor is in the first instance directed at determining the cause of the pallor and begins with a thorough history and physical examination, in particular, elucidating the onset and tempo of progression of visual loss and the presence of other neurological or systemic symptoms and signs.

Some of the causes of such optic neuropathy also cause significant morbidity or mortality. Examples of these are intracranial tumours, infections and inflammations. It is essential to sufficiently investigate optic disc pallor to exclude these.

Optic Disc Cupping

When faced with a cupped disc, it is essential to exclude glaucoma as a cause (see Chapter 4 on "Glaucoma"). Other optic neuropathies may uncommonly cause disc cupping, and should be considered as part of the differentials. In addition, if the patient has normal optic nerve function, which remains static over time, with no change in the optic disc appearance, this may represent physiological cupping.

Clinical Case: Examples of Optic Neuropathies

Optic Neuritis

A 28-year-old woman presents with right eye blurring of vision for 2–3 days. This is associated with a mild ache on eye movements, and she reports that the apple she was eating did not appear as red when seen with the right eye compared with her left eye. Her visual acuity is 6/24 on the right and 6/6 on the left. There is a right RAPD and she can only read 3 of 15 plates on the Ishihara charts. Confrontation visual fields reveals a central visual field defect. Figure 9.5 shows the optic nerve appearance and corresponding MRI scans of the orbits. The left eye is normal on examination.

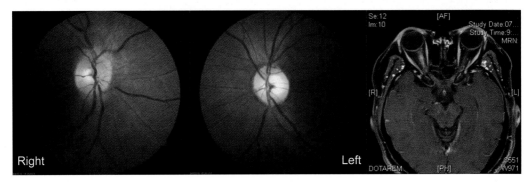

Fig. 9.5. Right optic disc swelling. Thickening and enhancement of the right optic nerve on T1 with contrast, axial cut of her MRI orbits and anterior visual pathway.

What is "Typical" (Demyelinating) Optic Neuritis?

Optic neuritis secondary to demyelination, which is typically associated with multiple sclerosis (MS)

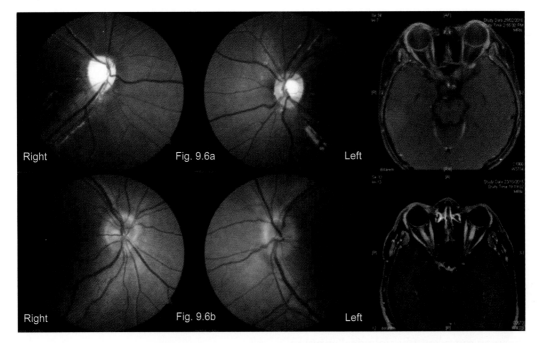

Fig. 9.6 (a,b). (a) Right pale disc from previous optic neuritis, with corresponding atrophy on imaging; b) bilateral swollen discs, which are thickened, and enhance with contrast on imaging, implying active inflammation of both optic nerves.

How else may Optic Neuritis present?

1. Optic neuritis maybe subclinical and present later as a pale disc (Fig. 9.6a)
2. Retrobulbar involvement, with absence of optic disc swelling
3. Bilateral disc involvement, with or without disc swelling (Fig. 9.6b)

What Other Diseases Cause Optic Neuritis?

The other common conditions that cause optic neuritis are Neuromyelitis Optica (NMO) and NMO Spectrum Disorder (NMOSD). Other autoimmune diseases such as sarcoidosis and systemic lupus erthymatosus can also cause an optic neuritis. Infections of the central nervous system such as tuberculosis or syphilis can give rise to a similar clinical picture. Such conditions should be suspected particularly when the optic neuritis is bilateral, painless, or associated with other neurological symptoms and signs

How should we Manage this Patient?

This patient can be offered intravenous corticosteroids (methylprednisolone) if there are no contraindications, as this has been shown to speed up visual recovery and improve contrast and visual defects

What is the Risk of developing Multiple Sclerosis?

The risk of multiple sclerosis depends on the presence of brain lesions in demyelinating optic neuritis. The presence of any brain lesion suggests the patient has a 72% risk of MS over 15 years compared to 15% if there are no brain lesions

Ischaemic Optic Neuropathy

A 65-year-old man presents with a sudden onset of blurring of vision of the right eye, which he noticed when he woke up in the morning. He has a past medical history of ischaemic heart disease, diabetes mellitus, hypertension, and smokes 1 packet of cigarettes a day. On examination, visual acuity is 6/12 on the right and 6/9 on the left. There is a right RAPD, and superior altitudinal defect on confrontational visual field testing of the right eye. His right optic disc is swollen, as seen in Fig. 9.7

What is the Diagnosis, and What Forms of this Condition are there? How do you tell them apart?

This patient has an ischaemic optic neuropathy (ION). This can affect the anterior portion of the optic disc, characterised by disc swelling, or the posterior portion, where the disc looks normal

Ischaemic optic neuropathy can be arteritic or non-arteritic (NA), and can affect the anterior of posterior portion of the nerve

Ophthalmologists use the term NAAION for non-arteritic anterior ischaemic optic neuropathy

What are the Risk Factors for NAAION?

- Ocular — small, crowded disc
- Systemic — hypertension, diabetes mellitus, hyperlipidaemia, ischaemic heart disease, carotid artery disease, sleep apnoea and smoking

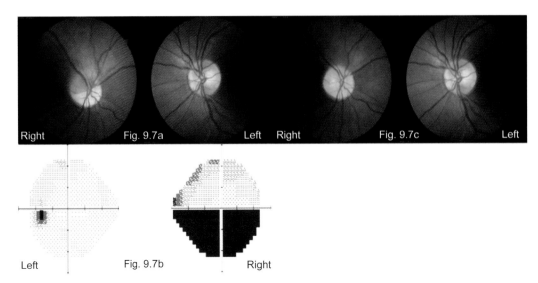

Fig. 9.7 (a-c). (a) Right optic disc swelling secondary to NAAION; (b) corresponding visual fields showing an inferior altitudinal defect; (c) 3 months later, right optic disc pallor is seen.

Table 9.2. Features of AAION and NAAION

	Arteritic Ischaemic Optic Neuropathy	Non-arteritic Ischaemic Optic Neuropathy
Patient	Typically >70 years old	Typically >50 years old,
Onset	Acute	Acute
History	May have features of giant cell arteritis — headaches, jaw claudication, scalp tenderness, hip and shoulder pain, and fever.	Risk factors as described above. No specific systemic symptoms.
Examination	Severe drop in visual acuity RAPD Any visual field defect Typically pale swelling of optic disc	Normal VA to HM RAPD Typically altitudinal field defect Swelling of optic disc
Investigations	Urgent ESR Temporal artery biopsy Coronary studies Pre-steroid work up	Blood pressure Fasting glucose, HbA1C Fasting lipids Sleep apnoea studies
Treatment	Urgent high dose intravenous steroids	Treatment of vascular risk factors

How should this Patient be Managed?

- Exclude arteritic AION
  - Take a good history for the symptoms described in Table 9.2
  - Test ESR, CRP, platelets (one or more of these three, particularly the ESR, is typically elevated)
- Modification of lifestyle — Smoking, Diet
- Investigate for risk factors — Fasting glucose and lipids, Blood pressure, studies for sleep apnoea

Raised Intracranial Pressure (ICP)

A 35-year-old woman presents with headaches for 2 months, associated with blurring of vision on waking. She has a background history of a brainstem tumour, which was treated with radiotherapy. Her visual acuity is 6/6 in both eyes, and there is no RAPD. Colour vision is normal. Optic discs, OCT of the disc and visual fields are shown in Fig. 9.8

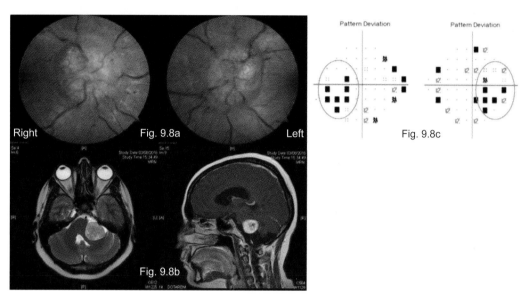

Fig. 9.8 (a-c). (a) Bilateral severely swollen discs; (b) neuroimaging showing a space occupying lesion compressing the fourth ventricle; (c) perimetry demonstrating enlarged blind spots (orange circles).

What are the Life-threatening Considerations in a patient with Bilateral Swollen Discs?

- Malignant hypertension
- Raised intracranial pressure
- Cerebral venous thrombosis

What Investigations should you Order?

- Urgent blood pressure check
- Urgent neuroimaging: MRI Brain and Magnetic Resonance Venogram (MRV)
- If above are normal, a Lumbar Puncture (LP) for opening pressure and CSF studies is indicated.

What are the Causes of Raised Intracranial Pressure?

- Space occupying lesions
- Infections / inflammations, e.g. meningitis
- Haemorrhage—spontaneous bleed or secondary to trauma
- Idiopathic

What is Idiopathic Intracranial Hypertension (IIH) / Pseudotumour Cerebri (PTC)?

IIH/PTC is a spectrum of disorders, with several associations (see below), which results in raised ICP, with no intracranial pathology found. These patients may present with headaches and/or disc swelling, with corresponding decrease in optic nerve function

What are the risk factors/associations for IIH/PTC?

- Obesity
- Hormones — hormonal imbalance from gynaecologic disease, medications (e.g. oral contraceptives)
- Medications—steroids (use or withdrawal), vitamin A, tetracycline

What are the diagnostic criteria for IIH/PTC (Modified Dandy Criteria)?

- Awake and alert patient
- Symptoms of raised ICP—headaches, blurring of vision
- Normal MRI
- Normal neurological examination except for Abducers Nerve (CN6 palsy)
- Raised opening pressures of >25 mm H_2O found on LP performed in the lateral decubitus position, with normal CSF composition.
- No other explanation for raised ICP

How are patients with IIH/PTC managed?

- Treat/remove any associations
- Lifestyle modifications—weight loss and management of other metabolic diseases
- Pain relief — analgesia for headaches
- Reduce ICP — acetazolamide, topiramate, surgical interventions (CSF shunts), and optic nerve sheath fenestration

> **Take home messages**
> Optic neuropathies can present as pale or swollen discs and could be classified as unilateral or bilateral.

9.2 Visual Field Defects

> **Learning Objectives**
> • To detect visual field defects on confrontational visual field.
> • To recognise patterns of monocular and binocular visual field defects and the site of the lesions causing these defects.

Detection of Visual Field (VF) Defects

Visual field examination should be performed for ALL patients who have visual complaints. Visual field defects may be monocular or binocular. While the cause of the visual field defect is not always apparent on ocular or neurologic examination, the pattern of the visual field defect is often suggestive of the site of insult to the visual pathway

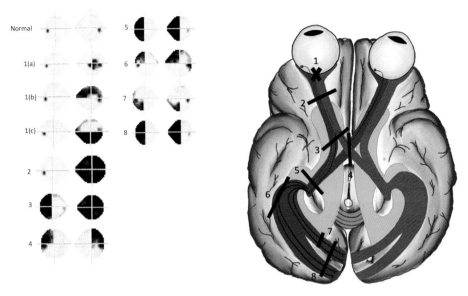

Fig. 9.9. Lesions of the visual pathway at various levels and their corresponding field defects.

Figure 9.9. illustrates the common visual field defects that one may encounter with lesions along the visual pathway. Table 9.3 summarises the common VF defects that we encounter in our practice and a guide to further investigations that we perform

Patients with visual field defects may have normal central visual acuity, and have non-specific complaints of general blurring, darkening of vision, presenting with unexplained falls or bumping into objects. Some others may be completely asymptomatic and found to have visual field defects when being screened for other conditions

In general, monocular field defects tend to suggest lesions in one eye or optic nerve, while certain patterns of binocular defects suggest lesions of the visual pathway beyond the optic nerves

Table 9.3. Examples of Commonly Encountered Visual Field Defects

Monocular visual field defects	Cause/site of lesion	Further Investigations (Guide)
1. Central scotoma 2. Inferior altitudinal defect 3. Arcuate defect arising from blind spot	1. Macula; optic nerve (e.g. optic neuritis) 2. Optic nerve (ischaemic optic neuropathy) 3. Optic nerve (glaucoma)	• Macula OCT • Fluorescein angiogram • OCT RNFL • MRI of the orbits and anterior visual pathway ± brain
Binocular visual field defects 1. Pattern of monocular visual loss, which presents bilaterally 2. Bitemporal hemianopia 3. Homonymous hemianopia 4. Homonymous superior quadrantanopia 5. Homonymous superior quadrantanopia	1. Bilateral optic neuropathies or retinopathies 2. Optic chiasm 3. Contralateral retrochiasmal visual pathway 4. Contralateral temporal lobe* 5. Contralateral parietal lobe* *Suggestive but not exclusive	MRI of the orbits and anterior visual pathway ± brain Lumbar puncture if indicated

Monocular Visual Field Defects

Monocular visual field defects are usually ocular in origin. However, at times, visual pathway disorders can present as monocular visual field defects either because they are asymmetrical, or because only the central visual fields were examined

When dealing with a monocular visual field defect, it is important to consider both optic neuropathies, as well as retinopathies (which include maculopathies) as differential diagnoses. Retinal causes of visual loss will be discussed in Chapter 6

Figure 9.10 shows a superior arcuate defect secondary to glaucomatous damage to the optic nerve

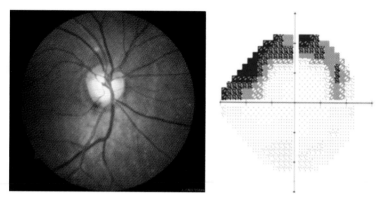

Fig. 9.10. Thinning of the optic nerve rim inferiorly with associated drance haemorrhage secondary to glaucoma.

Binocular Visual Field Defects

Binocular visual field defects can occur as a result of bilateral optic neuropathies or retinopathies (Fig. 9.11) or from a lesion anywhere along the visual pathway from the optic chiasm to the occipital lobe. Because of the way the fibres of the visual pathway are arranged, visual field defects tend to be more congruous if the lesion is more posterior. For example, an occipital lobe lesion (Fig. 9.12) will give rise to a visual field defect that is more congruous than that of a pre-geniculate optic tract lesion

As patients may report blurring of vision as their chief complaint, it is crucial to enquire if they occluded one eye to determine the side of blurring. More often than not, hemianopias or quadrantanopias may be thought to be blurring of vision of side of the visual field defect

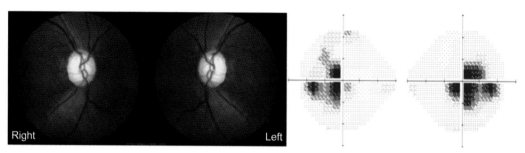

Fig. 9.11. Bilateral optic disc cupping and temporal pallor, with corresponding cecocentral visual field defects, likely secondary to hereditary optic neuropathy.

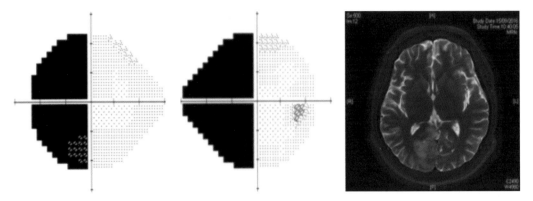

Fig. 9.12. Congruous homonymous hemianopia secondary to occipital lobe infarction.

Clinical Case Examples of Visual Field Defects

Bitemporal Hemianopia

A 28-year-old man was referred after he sustained an injury from bumping into objects. He was otherwise asymptomatic but on further questioning revealed that he had breast enlargement. His visual acuity was 6/6 bilaterally and he had normal colour vision. There was no RAPD. On clinical examination, he was found to have bow tie pallor of his optic discs (Fig. 9.13), and a bitemporal hemianopia. MRI scan showed a pituitary macroadenoma, compressing on the optic chiasm (Fig. 9.14)

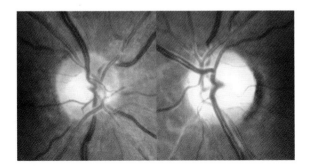

Fig. 9.13. Bow-tie optic disc pallor, which is more evident on the left.

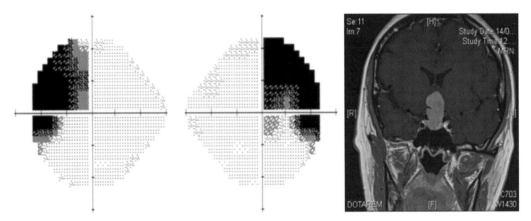

Fig. 9.14. Bitemporal hemianopia secondary to a pituitary macroadenoma.

What Other Investigations should be Performed?

In addition to neuroimaging, investigation of the pituitary hormones should be performed.

How should you Manage patients with Pituitary Adenomas?

- Co-manage with endocrinologist and neurosurgeon
- Medical treatment (individualised) — hormone supplements, carbagoline or bromocriptine (for prolactinoma)
- Surgical intervention is indicated if there is evidence of compressive optic neuropathy, progressive enlargement of tumour and/or invasion of the cavernous sinus

Homonymous Hemianopia

A 70-year-old Chinese man, with a background of diabetes mellitus and hypertension, presented with right sided blurring of vision for 2 days. He was still able drive and read the newspapers. Visual acuities were 6/6 in either eye, and the ocular examination was unremarkable apart from age related cataracts. His colour vision and pupil examination were normal, and he was found to have right homonymous hemianopia on visual field testing. Urgent neuroimaging confirmed the presence of a stroke of the left occipital lobe (Fig. 9.15)

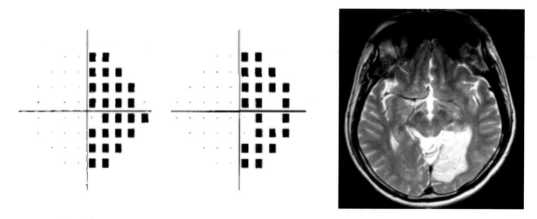

Fig. 9.15. Macular sparing right homonymous hemianopia secondary to a left occipital infarct.

How will you Manage this Patient?

- Determine risk factors for stroke — investigate for hypertension, diabetes mellitus, hyperlipidaemia and sources of emboli
- Co-manage with neurologist
- Treat underlying risk factors

Take home messages

The pattern of visual field defect can help to localise the lesion.

9.3 Ocular Motility Disorders

Learning Objectives
• Understand the innervation of the extraocular muscles and identify motility disorders (limitations).
• Understand the use of cover test in the context of strabismus resulting from neuro-ophthalmic disease.
• Recognize common patterns of ocular motility abnormalities.

History

Ocular motility disorders frequently present with diplopia. However, some patients may not complain of any visual symptoms, and some may report slight blurring of vision. When faced with a patient who has diplopia, it is important to determine the following:

The important details to determine in the evaluation of a patient with diplopia are:
• Is the diplopia monocular or binocular? (Table 9.4)

• Is the diplopia vertical, horizontal or oblique (torsional)? This refers to the location and orientation of the second image

• Is the diplopia the same in all directions of gaze? This refers to the separation and orientation of the images

• Is the diplopia constant or intermittent?

• Has the diplopia been static since onset or progressive?

Table 9.4. Causes of Diplopia

Monocular	Binocular		
Tends to be ocular in nature	Paretic		Restrictive
	Supranuclear	Nuclear/Infranuclear/NMJ/Muscle	1. Thyroid eye disease
1. Cornea*		1. Cranial nerve palsies (Single/ Multiple)	
2. Lens*			2. Orbital inflammatory disease
3. Macula		2. Myasthenia gravis	
4. Cerebral polyopia (rare)		3. Myopathies	3. Orbital wall fractures

*Monocular diplopia from disturbances in the optical media typically resolves when looking through a pinhole.

Ocular Motility Examination

The ocular motility examination is directed at elucidating the site and cause of the ocular motility defect. It begins with determining if there is any limitation in ocular motility, whether it is restrictive or paretic, and the nerve(s) and/or muscle(s) involved. The innervation of the extraocular muscles is shown in Table 9.5

The basic eye movement examination consists of examining pursuit (slow) movements to determine the range (extent) of eye movements into the different positions of gaze. The eyes are first observed in the primary position (looking straight ahead) using the corneal light reflex (Hirschberg test) to determine relative position of the eyes. The patient is then asked to track a target into the nine cardinal positions of gaze (including primary position)

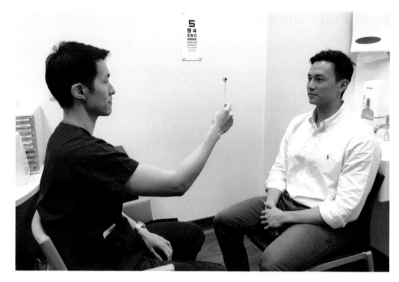

Fig. 9.16a. Performing the ocular motility examination with an accommodative target.

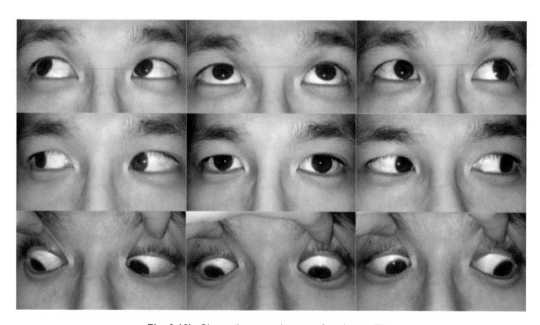

Fig. 9.16b. Shows the normal range of ocular motility.

to determine how far the eyes move into each of those positions. Figure 9.16 shows a normal ocular motility examination

Further Eye Mmovement Testing includes:

- Saccadic (fast) eye movements
- Cover test in the different gaze positions (primary position, right, left, up and down-gaze as well as right and left head tilts). The alternate cover test dissociates the eyes and allows for small angles of deviation to be detected by the examiner. This allows subtle ocular motility defects to be elucidated. The angle of deviation can also be measured using prisms, and this is important for diagnosis and follow up (See Chapter 8 on "Paediatric Ophthalmology")

Table 9.5. Innervation of and Movements Produced by the Extraocular Muscles

	Primary Action	Secondary Action	Tertiary Action	Innervation
Medial rectus	Adduction	-	-	3rd (oculomotor) cranial nerve
Lateral rectus	Abduction	-	-	6th (abducens) cranial nerve
Superior rectus	Elevation	Intorsion	Adduction	3rd (oculomotor) cranial nerve
Inferior rectus	Depression	Extorsion	Adduction	3rd (oculomotor) cranial nerve
Superior oblique	Intorsion	Depression	Abduction	4th (trochlear) cranial nerve
Inferior oblique	Extorsion	Elevation	Abduction	3rd (oculomotor) cranial nerve

Clinical Case Examples of Ocular Motility Disorders

Oculomotor Nerve Palsy

A 45-year-old man with a past medical history of diabetes mellitus, hypertension and hyperlipidaemia presented acutely with ptosis and binocular diplopia. His eye movements in 9 positions of gaze (Fig. 9.17) are shown below. There was no anisocoria, and the remainder of the ocular examination, including optic nerve function was otherwise normal

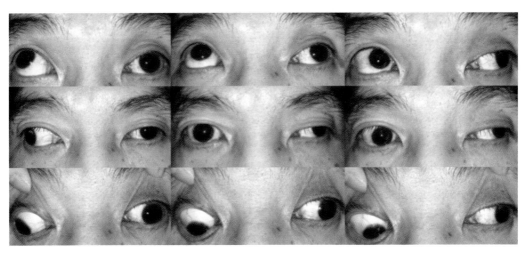

Fig. 9.17. Ocular motility.

What is the Diagnosis?

Partial, pupil-sparing oculomotor nerve palsy (CN3 Palsy)

Should this Patient have Neuroimaging?

Yes. Urgent neuroimaging in the form of MRI brain with contrast and MR angiogram should be performed. This patient may have an evolving CN3 Palsy, which could still be due to a compressive lesion, such as a posterior communicating artery aneurysm

In what Situation can this be Observed?

The only third nerve palsy that can be closely monitored without initial neuroimaging is one that is painless, complete (complete ptosis, limitation of eye movements in all directions except abduction), pupil-sparing and occurring in a patient >50 years of age who has appropriate vascular risk factors

Abducens Nerve Palsy

A 63-year-old woman, with background history of diabetes mellitus and hypertension, presents with a 2-day history of acute, binocular, horizontal diplopia. Her visual acuity is 6/6 bilaterally and pupillary examination is unremarkable. Her range of eye movements is shown in Fig. 9.18

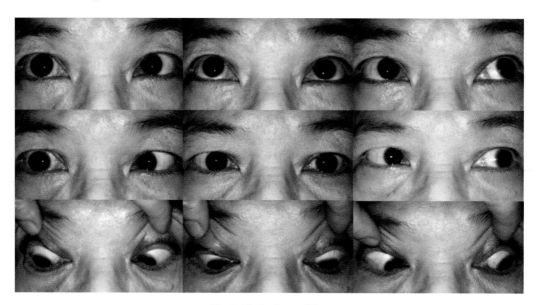

Fig. 9.18. Ocular motility.

What are the Possible Causes of an Abduction Deficit?

Paretic	Restrictive
Abducens nerve palsy	Medial wall fractures
Myasthenia gravis	Thyroid eye disease
Miller fisher syndrome	Muscle fibrosis from longstanding palsy

What does this patient have? What else is Important in her Examination?

- Right ischaemic abducens nerve palsy (CN6 palsy)

- CN6 palsy maybe a false localising sign in raised intracranial pressure. All patients with a CN6 palsy should have a dilated fundus examination to exclude optic disc(s) swelling secondary to raised ICP

How should she be Managed?

- Co-manage ischaemic risk factors with the internist

- Conservative management as there is a good chance of spontaneous recovery with monocular occlusion or prisms for relief of diplopia.

- Surgery should only be considered after AT LEAST 6 months of observation, with stable prism cover test measurements

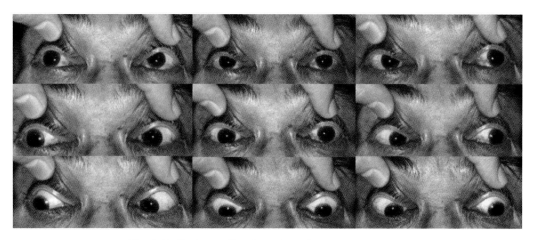

Fig. 9.19. Ocular motility of a patient with myasthenia gravis.

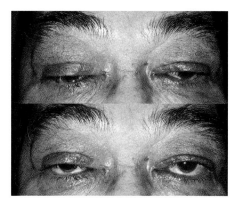

Fig. 9.20. Pre- and post ice pack test.

Myasthenia Gravis

A 60-year-old man presents with 1–2 months history of variable ptosis, which worsens in the evenings, and fluctuating diplopia throughout the day. Ocular examination reveals cataract and limitation of eye movements in all directions of gaze (Fig. 9.19). In addition, there is improvement of his ptosis by >2 mm after an ice pack test (Fig. 9.20)

What are the Differential Diagnoses?

- Myasthenia gravis
- Multiple cranial nerve palsies
- Myopathies, e.g. myotonic dystrophy, chronic progressive external ophthalmoplegia

What is the Pathology in Myasthenia Gravis (MG)?

The muscle weakness that occurs in MG is secondary to antibodies at the neuromuscular junction (NMJ), which interfere with normal interaction between acetylcholine and its receptors (Fig. 9.21).

How is the Diagnosis of Myasthenia Gravis made?

- Clinical — ice pack test, neostigmine test, edrophonium test
- Biochemical — anti-acetylcholine receptor antibody, anti-muscle specific kinase antibody

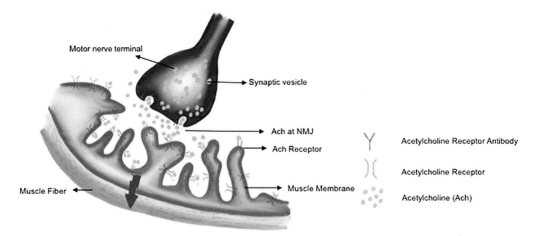

Fig. 9.21a. Normal neuromuscular junction (NMJ). Ach release and its interaction with nicotinic receptors on the muscle membrane.

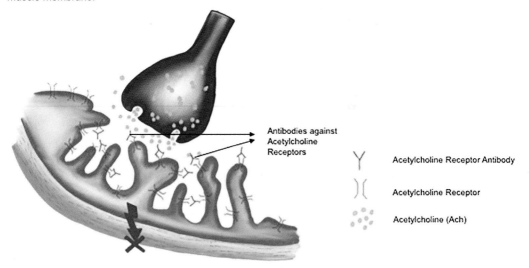

Fig. 9.21b. NMJ in myasthenia gravis. In myasthenia gravis, the normal interaction between the Ach and its receptors is affected by presence of antibodies, which compete with Ach to bind with the receptors, causing weakness of muscle contraction.

- Electrophysiology — single-fibre electromyogram and repetitive nerve stimulation
- Imaging (Supporting test) — in patients with myasthenia, a CT thorax should be performed to exclude a thymoma

What is the Treatment of Myasthenia?

- Anti-cholinesterase, e.g. pyridostigmine
- Corticosteroids and / or steroid-sparing agents
- Thymectomy (if there is a thymoma)
- Plasmapheresis and intravenous immunoglobulin (typically for generalised myasthenia or myasthenic crisis)

Take home messages

Consider myasthenia gravis in all ocular motility deficits.

9.4 Pupillary Abnormalities

Learning Objectives
- To be able to perform complete examination of the pupils.
- To appreciate the various abnormalities in relation to afferent and efferent pathway disorders.

History

Pupillary abnormalities may be discovered incidentally by the patient, family member, or during an ocular examination. At times, pupil abnormalities present as part of another ophthalmic problem that was brought to attention, for example, in the case of a pupil involving CN3 palsy

Important questions to ask in the history depend on the type of pupillary abnormality found. In addition, questions pertaining to general health, existing comorbities, medication (topical and systemic) as well as a history of trauma are important in all patients. More specific questions are listed below

Anisocoria

- How was it noticed?
- Any pain — including headache, neck pain
- History of Trauma?
- Use of medications
- Presence of other symptoms including diplopia (which might suggest an oculomotor nerve palsy), limb weakness or numbness?

Relative Afferent Pupillary Defect (RAPD)

- Any preceding visual loss? (Important to examine the optic nerve function)
- Neurological deficits

Light-near Dissociation

- History of diabetes mellitus
- Sexual history / known history of syphilis or herpetic infection
- Others: Alcohol consumption, recent illness

Case Example of Pupillary Abnormality

Horner's Syndrome

A 68-year-old Chinese man complains of right sided mild ptosis. He also has a background history of weight loss and epistaxis. He had no prior history of eyelid trauma, cataract surgery or contact lens use and he denied use of any topical medications. Visual acuity was 6/9 bilaterally, and apart from nuclear sclerotic cataracts, examination of the anterior and posterior segments was unremarkable. He was noted to have anisocoria, which was worse in the dark. Apraclonidine eye drops reversed the anisocoria (Fig. 9.22)

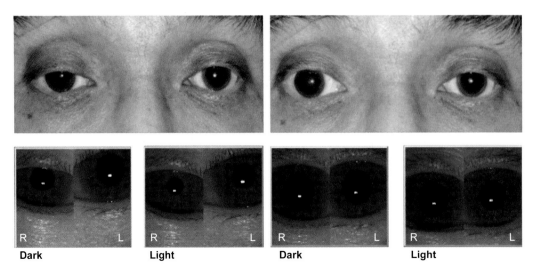

| Dark | Light | Dark | Light |

Fig. 9.22. Pre- and post apraclonidine test, demonstrating right eyelid elevation and reversal of anisocoria.

What is Horner's Syndrome?

Horner's syndrome refers to the constellation of findings (partial ptosis, miosis and/or anhidrosis) resulting from a lesion affecting any part of the sympathetic pathway

In this patient, it was secondary to nasopharyngeal carcinoma, which invaded the cavernous sinus

What are the Potential Life-threatening Causes of Horner's Syndrome?

- Intracranial pathology — strokes, compressive lesions
- Neck pathology — Pancoast tumour, enlarged thyroid, lymphadenopathy, trauma
- Vascular — carotid artery dissection, cavernous sinus infiltration

How do you Diagnose Horner's Syndrome?

- Confirmatory tests — Cocaine test, Apraclonidine test
- Localisation tests — Hydroxyamphetamine test, Phenylephine text
- Appropriate imaging

Take home messages

Horner's syndrome comprises of a triad of partial ptosis, miosis and anhidrosis.

References

1. American Academy of Ophthalmology, *Neuro-ophthalmology* **87**: 2014-2015.

2. Digre KB, *et al.* (2001) "Idiopathic intracranial hypertension (pseudotumor cerebri): A reappraisal." *Neurologist* **7**: 2–67.

3. Optic Neuritis Study Group. (2008) Visual function 15 years after optic neuritis: a final follow-up report from the optic neuritis treatment trial. *Ophthalmology* **115**(6): 1079–1082 e5.

4. Walsh and Hoyt's *Clinical Neuro-ophthalmology: The Essentials*, 2nd ed.. Nuclear and Infranuclear Ocular Motility Disorders Chapter 18, page 391.

5. Wingerchuck DM, *et al.* (2006) Revised diagnostic criteria for neuromyelitis optica. *Neurology* **66**(10):1485–1489.

Chapter 10

PRINCIPLES AND PRACTICE OF LOW VISION REHABILITATION

Learning Objectives
- Understand the role of low vision care in ophthalmology.
- Identify patients with low vision.
- Understand the functional impact of low vision.
- Understand low vision evaluation and management.
- Refer patient for low vision rehabilitation services.

The number of elderly living with vision loss will increase over the decades with the aging population and increasing longevity in Singapore and globally. Therefore, understanding the principles of low vision care and practice is critical and relevant.

10.1 What is Low Vision?

Low vision is vision impairment that is not corrected by standard eyeglasses, or by medical or surgical treatment. It may result from many different ocular and neurological disorders

A person with low vision is one who has:
- An impairment of visual functioning even after treatment and/or standard refraction correction
- A visual acuity of less than 6/18 to light perception
- A visual field of less than 10° from the point of fixation, but who
- Uses or is potentially able to use, vision for the planning and/or execution of a task

Lighthouse International revised this definition of visual impairment that included aspects of functioning:

Functional visual impairment is a significant limitation of visual capability resulting from disease, trauma or congenital condition which cannot be fully ameliorated by standard refractive correction, medication or surgery, and is manifested by one of the following:
- Insufficient visual resolution (worse than 6/12 in the better eye with best correction of ametropia)
- Inadequate field of vision (20° or worse along the widest meridian in the eye with the more intact central field; homonymous hemianopia)

- Reduced peak contrast sensitivity (<1.7 log CS binocularly)
- Insufficient visual resolution or peak contrast sensitivity at high or low luminances within the range typically encountered in everyday life

This expanded definition takes a functional perspective, and compels us to consider any patient who has difficulty performing a visual task as potentially in need of low vision care and rehabilitation

The American Academy of Ophthalmology's Smartsight Model of Vision Rehabilitation similarly adopts this functional definition of low vision and calls for ophthalmologists to refer patients with low vision for rehabilitation at two levels

- Level 1 asks all ophthalmologists who see patients with less than 6/12 visual acuity in the better eye, contrast sensitivity loss, scotoma, or field loss to "recognise" and "respond" by assuring patients that much can be offered with rehabilitation
- Level 2 incorporates comprehensive multidisciplinary vision rehabilitation care process as part of the continuum of ophthalmic care

10.2 Functional Impact of Low Vision

In low vision care, it is crucial to understanding pathology from a functional perspective and explains visual deficits and complaints. The pathological process correlates with the patient's functional status. It also influences management decisions, the types of optical aids and vision rehabilitation services needed, and the patient's ability to respond to those interventions

Faye *et al.* classified three types of visual deficits based on the effects of functional vision, which is paramount when approaching the patient with low vision – cloudy media (Fig. 10.1), central field deficit (Fig. 10.2) and peripheral field deficit (Fig. 10.3)

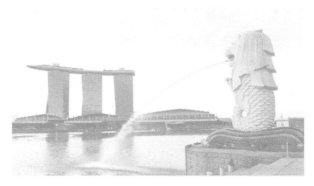

Fig. 10.1. Cloudy media.

Cloudy Media

Common Aetiology
- Corneal scars, dystrophy and oedema
- Pupil/iris atrophy, polycoria and iridectomy
- Inoperable cataract
- Vitreous inflammation and haemorrhage

Functional Implications

- Blurred vision for distance and near tasks
- Faded colours
- Glare disability
- Reduced contrast sensitivity

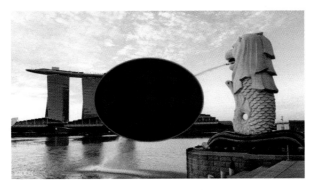

Fig. 10.2. Central field deficit.

Central Field Deficit

Common Aetiology

- Age-related macular degeneration
- Macular scar and ischaemia

Functional Implications

- Varies depending on number, size, location and density of scotoma
- Reduced central vision for distance, intermediate and near tasks; reading and facial recognition
- Reduced retinal illuminance

Peripheral Field Deficit

Common Aetiology

- Advanced glaucoma

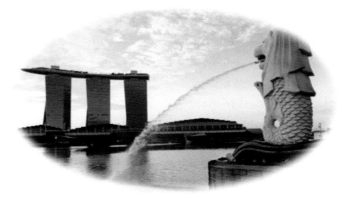

Fig. 10.3. Peripheral field deficit.

- Retinitis pigmentosa
- Neurologic (stroke, tumours)

Functional Implications

- Mobility in unfamiliar environments
- Anxiety and bumping into peripheral objects
- Mobility at night and under poor illumination
- Locating objects

Low Vision Evaluation

The low vision evaluation takes a functional and clinical approach to optimise patient performance in daily living tasks and include the following components:

- History
- Visual acuity and refraction
- Visual field testing
- Contrast sensitivity function
- Magnification evaluation

History

The history aims to uncover the patient's chief complaint and functional loss. Therefore, it is important to think not just in terms of anatomical lesions, but also in terms of the patient's loss of ability to perform daily living tasks. The history covers the following aspects:

- Chief complaint
- Visual/ocular history
- General health review
- Activities of daily living
- Lifestyle, education and career history
- Social history and support systems
- Psycho-social issues, adjustment and coping
- Functional and task-related history
- Priorities and goals of rehabilitation

Visual Acuity and Refraction

Visual acuity and refraction are performed to establish the patient's residual vision and to determine visual disability. Assessing visual acuity and refraction is critical to:

- Monitor the effect, progression and treatment of eye diseases
- Determine the magnification of optical low vision aids for reading
- Verify a patient's visual fitness to drive
- Classify patients as "legally blind" for assistance schemes, support services, benefits and exemptions

The Early Treatment Diabetic Retinopathy Study (ETDRS) chart is widely used in low vision assessment as it incorporates accepted principles of chart design (Fig. 10.4)

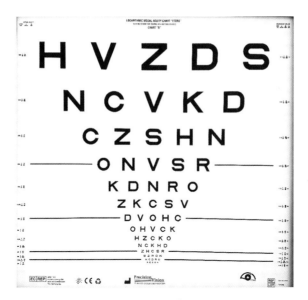

Fig. 10.4. ETDRS chart.

Visual Field Testing

Perimetry, or visual field testing aims to evaluate the depth and breadth of a patient's field of view. For absolute peripheral field defect, dynamic visual field testing such as a Tangent screen or Goldmann perimetry is useful (Fig. 10.5). For central field defect, threshold testing such as the Humphrey visual field analyser or California Central Field Test is more appropriate (Fig. 10.6). The purpose of undertaking visual field testing in low vision is to explain the nature of disability described or noted by the patient

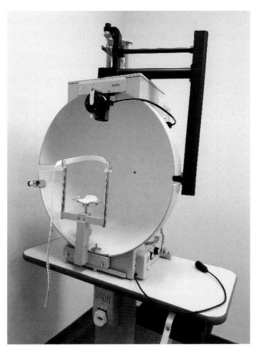

Fig. 10.5. Goldmann perimeter.

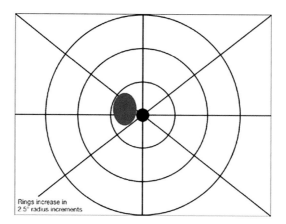

Fig. 10.6. California Central Field Test.

A recent development in low vision evaluation is assessment of scotomas (blind spots within the visual field) and training patients to use healthy retinal areas to optimise viewing Visual field testing is important for the following reasons:

- Provide objective information about scotomas and correlate with poor task performance
- Show patterns of peripheral field loss for the indication of orientation and mobility training and rehabilitation planning
- Follow disease progression and explain functional visual change that does not correlate with acuity or contrast test

Contrast Sensitivity Function

Contrast sensitivity function is critical in activities such as face recognition and navigating steps. The Pelli-Robson Chart (Fig. 10.7) is commonly used to assess contrast sensitivity. This test is valuable to help the patient gain greater understanding of the nature of their visual impairment and why certain adaptive strategies can be adopted to optimise vision

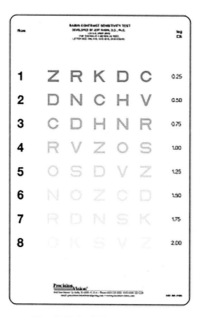

Fig. 10.7. Pelli-Robson chart.

Contrast sensitivity is useful for:

- Determining magnification need
- Assessing ability to use optical low vision aids
- Determining optimal illumination level to maximise vision
- Monitoring disease progression
- Understanding overall functioning of the patient and plan rehabilitative strategies

Magnification Evaluation

The primary management for low vision is to optimise residual vision through magnification — the process of optically enlarging the retinal image with an optical device. After a low vision evaluation and complete assessment of the patient's needs and visual abilities, an optical device is prescribed to enhance function and critical tasks in everyday life, education and work. Magnification can be achieved using four different methods:

- Relative size magnification
- Relative distance (approach) magnification
- Angular magnification
- Electronic magnification

Relative size magnification involves physically enlarging texts or using large print devices (Fig. 10.8)

Relative distance magnification is achieved by bringing objects closer (approaching) to the eyes, and focussing the image with a magnifier (Fig. 10.9)

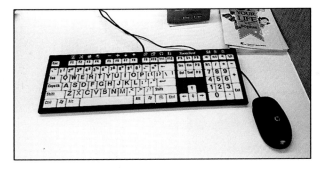

Fig. 10.8. Large keyboard.

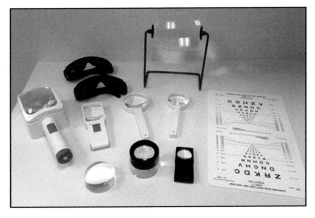

Fig. 10.9. Optical devices.

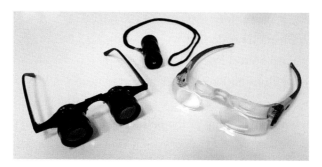

Fig. 10.10. Binocular spectacles and telescope.

Angular magnification is enlargement when the patient looks through a telescopic device (Fig. 10.10)

Electronic magnification combines relative size and relative distance magnification, with the use of electronic magnification devices (Fig. 10.11)

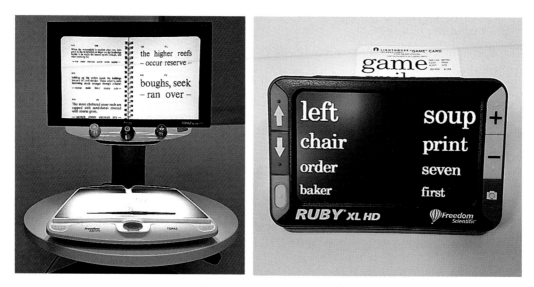

Fig. 10.11. Desktop and portable electronic magnifier.

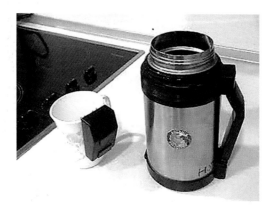

Fig. 10.12. Liquid level indicator.

Visual Substitution

When visual impairment progresses to a severe stage, optical devices may be inappropriate or impractical. At this stage, patients is taught to compensate with their other senses such as touch, hearing, taste, and smell by using sensorial devices such as Braille, tactile watches, talking clocks, liquid level indicators and audio books (Fig. 10.12)

Comprehensive Low Vision Rehabilitation

Comprehensive low vision care and rehabilitation involves a team-based, multidisciplinary and integrated approach, and include:

- Occupational therapy — training the patient to perform activities of daily living
- Orientation and mobility training — teaching navigation skills
- Counselling and mental health services
- Career and assistive technology services

Take home messages

- Low vision rehabilitation plays a significant role in minimising disability and improving quality of life for patients with low vision.
- All ophthalmic professionals involved in clinical practice have a responsibility to be informed about it and to refer patients appropriately and seamlessly.

References

1. American Academy of Ophthalmology. Vision Rehabilitation Committee. (2013) *Preferred Practice Pattern® Guidelines. Vision Rehabilitation for Adults.* San Francisco, CA: American Academy of Ophthalmology.

2. Arditi A, Rosenthal B. (1996) *Developing an Objective Definition of Visual Impairment.* New York: Arlene R. Gordon Research Institute, The Lighthouse Inc.

3. Colenbrander A. (2010) Assessment of functional vision and its rehabilitation. *Acta Ophthalmol* **88**:163–173.

4. Colenbrander A, Goodwin L, Fletcher DC. (2007) Vision rehabilitation and AMD. *Int Ophthalmol Clin* **47**:139–148.

5. Dickinson C. (1998) *Low Vision: Principles and Practice.* Oxford: Butterworth-Heinemann.

6. Faye EE. (1976) *Clinical Low Vision*, 1st ed.. New York: Little Brown and Company.

7. Fletcher DC, Schuchard RA. (1997) Preferred retinal loci relationship to macular scotomas in a low vision population. *Ophthalmology* **104**:632–638.

8. Jackson AJ, Wolffsohn JS. (2007) *Low Vision Manual.* Philadelphia, USA: Butterworth-Heinemann.

9. Markowitz S. (2006) Principles of modern low vision rehabilitation. *Can J Ophthalmol* **41**:289–312.

10. National Research Council, National Academy of Sciences. (1980) Recommended standard procedures for the clinical measurement and specification of visual acuity. *Adv Ophthalmol* **41**:103–148.

11. Pelli DG, Robson JG, Wilkins AJ. (1988) The design of a new letter chart for measuring contrast sensitivity. *Clin Vis Sci* **2**:187–199.

12. Whittaker SG, Scheiman M, Sokol-McKay DA. (2016) *Low Vision Rehabilitation. A Guide for Occupational Therapists*, 2nd ed.. New Jersey, USA: Slack Incorporated.

13. World Health Organization. (1993) *Management of Low Vision in Children*. Geneva, Switzerland: World Health Organization.

Chapter 11

CLINICAL APPROACHES

11.1 Approach to Leukocoria

Presenting Complaint:
- Age of onset
  - Bilateral RB → 1 year
  - Unilateral RB → 2 years
- Duration of white reflex
  - From birth → congenital causes, e.g. PFV
  - Acquired later on eg. RB
- Other symptoms
  - Pain, redness → RB with anterior segment involvement
  - Strabismus → RB, cataract

Past medical / ocular history:
- Premature birth → ROP
- Trauma → cataract
- Infections e.g. TORCH → Toxoplasmosis, cataract
- Exposure to pets → Toxoplasmosis

Family History:
- Present → RB, FEVR, coloboma

Legend: AC = anterior chamber; FEVR = familial exudative vitreoretinopathy; IOP = intraocular pressure; PFV = persistent fetal vasculature; RB = retinoblastoma; ROP = retinopathy of prematurity; RD = retinal detachment; TORCH = **t**oxoplasmosis, **o**ther (syphilis, Varicella zoster, parvovirus B19), **r**ubella, **c**ytomegalovirus, **h**erpes infections

WHITE PUPILLARY REFLEX noticed on –
- Flash photography
- Observation by family members
- Examination of the red reflex

CLINICAL EXAMINATION

CHARACTERISTICS
Laterality:
- Unilateral → RB, Coats', PFV, toxocariasis
- Bilateral → RB, FEVR, ROP

Colour of reflex:
- White → RB
- Yellow → exudates, RD, Coats'
- Blue/Gray → cataract

IOP:
- High IOP → could be secondary to anterior segment neovascularisation in RB/Coats'
- Strabismus present?
- Commonly present in RB, cataract

ANTERIOR SEGMENT
- Small eye with shallow AC → PFV
- Iris coloboma → choroidal coloboma
- Inflammation or neovascularisation in AC → RB, Coats', longstanding RD
- Crystalline cholesterol deposits in AC → Coats
- Lens opacity → cataract, PFV

- B scan Ultrasonography —
  - Low reflectivity → Coats', RD, toxocariasis
  - High internal acoustic reflectivity → RB (due to calcium)
  - Persistent hyaloid remnants → PFV
- Fundus fluorescein angiography (FFA) –
  - Retinal telangiectasia "light bulbs" → Coats'
  - Rapid homogenous hyperfluorescence → RB
  - Reticular hyperfluorescence → toxocariasis
  - Peripheral avascular zone → ROP, FEVR
- Magnetic resonance imaging (MRI) –
  - RB → evaluate pineal gland
- Blood serology —
  - Toxocariasis, TORCH infections
- Genetic testing —
  - Important for genetic counselling in patients with RB, FEVR, Coats

POSTERIOR SEGMENT
- Vitreous —
  - Seeding → RB
  - Vitritis → Toxocariasis
  - Persistent hyaloid canal → PFV
- Optic disc –
  - Excavation → morning glory disc anomaly, optic disc coloboma
  - Bergmeister papilla → PFV
- Blood vessels
  - Uniformly dilated/tortuous → RB
  - Irregular saccular dilation → Coats'

11.2 Clinical Pathway for Chronic Visual Loss

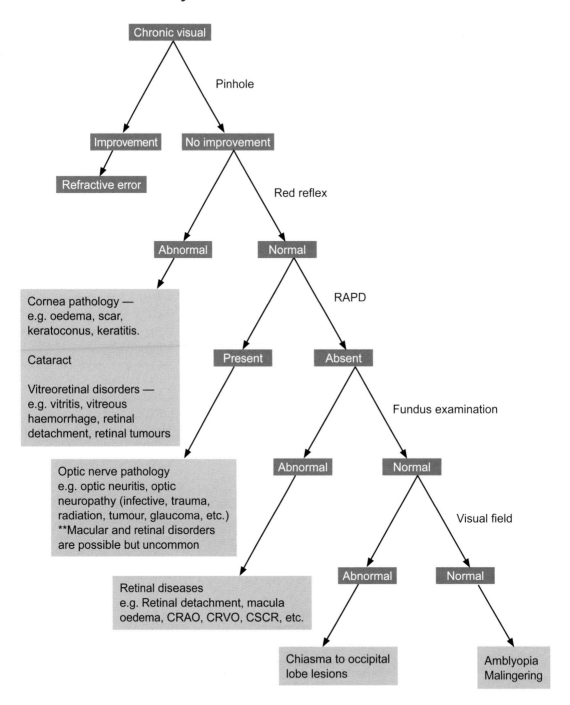

Abbreviations:
RAPD - Relative Afferent Pupillary Defect
CRAO - Central Retinal Artery Occlusion
CRVO -Central Retina Vein Occlusion
CSCR - Central Serous Chorioretinopathy

11.3 Clinical Pathway for Acute Visual Loss

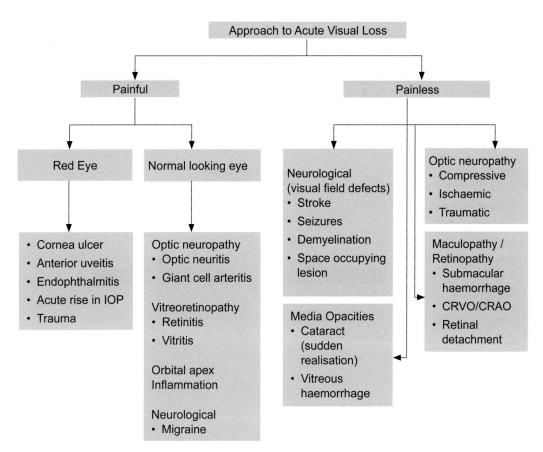

11.4 Diagnostic Flowchart in an Acute Red Eye

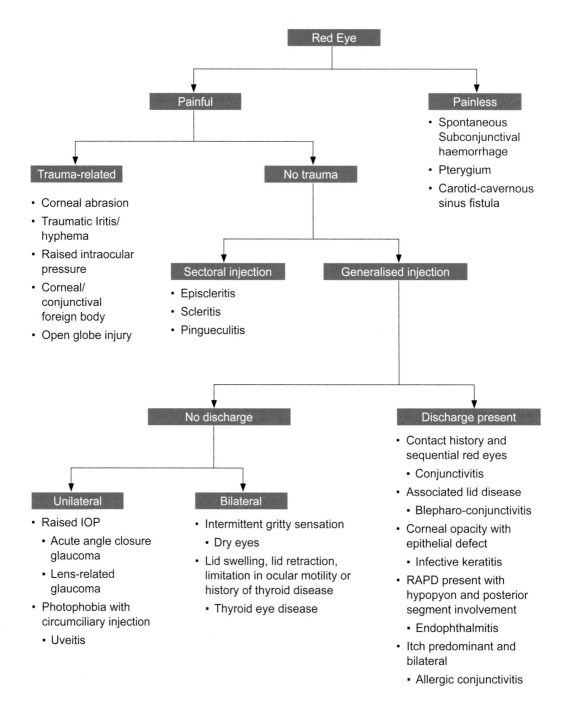

Red Eye

Painful

Painless
- Spontaneous Subconjunctival haemorrhage
- Pterygium
- Carotid-cavernous sinus fistula

Trauma-related
- Corneal abrasion
- Traumatic Iritis/ hyphema
- Raised intraocular pressure
- Corneal/ conjunctival foreign body
- Open globe injury

No trauma

Sectoral injection
- Episcleritis
- Scleritis
- Pingueculitis

Generalised injection

No discharge

Discharge present
- Contact history and sequential red eyes
  - Conjunctivitis
- Associated lid disease
  - Blepharo-conjunctivitis
- Corneal opacity with epithelial defect
  - Infective keratitis
- RAPD present with hypopyon and posterior segment involvement
  - Endophthalmitis
- Itch predominant and bilateral
  - Allergic conjunctivitis

Unilateral
- Raised IOP
  - Acute angle closure glaucoma
  - Lens-related glaucoma
- Photophobia with circumciliary injection
  - Uveitis

Bilateral
- Intermittent gritty sensation
  - Dry eyes
- Lid swelling, lid retraction, limitation in ocular motility or history of thyroid disease
  - Thyroid eye disease

11.5 Neuro-ophthalmology Approaches

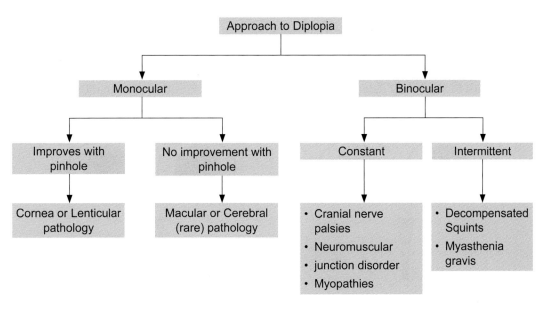

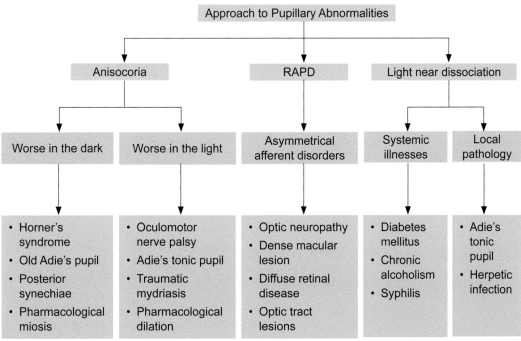

11.6 Pupil Examination

There are several steps involved in completing the pupil examination (Figs. 11.1a and 11.1b).

Examination of Pupil Size (testing for anisocoria) (Fig.s 11.1a and b)

Diffuse illumination of both eyes with a torch

Diffuse illumination is performed in the light, as Asian eyes typically have dark iris, making it difficult to accurately determine pupil size without background illumination

The light should not obstruct the visual axis.

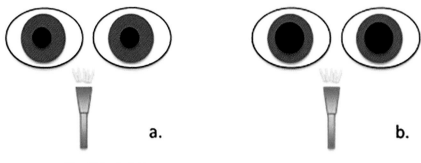

Fig. 11.1a. In light.   **Fig. 11.1b.** In the dark.

Direct and Consensual Light Reflex (Figs. 11.1c-i to 11.1c-iii)

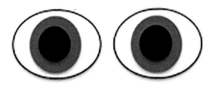

c-i.

Fig. 11.1c-i. Demonstrates normal pupils in the dark.

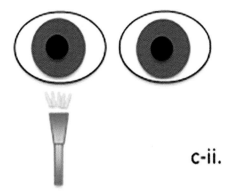

c-ii.

Fig. 11.1c-ii. On direct stimulation of a normal pupil, with a bright, focussed light source, the pupil constricts briskly.

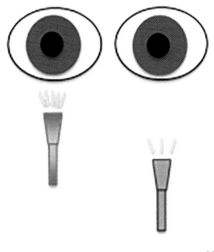

c-iii.

Fig. 11.1c-iii. Using a dim light (grey torch), the other pupil can be seen to react briskly as well, owing to a normal consensual light response.

Swinging Torchlight Test (Figs. 11.1d-i to 11.1d-iv demonstrate how a Relative Afferent Pupillary Defect is found on this test)

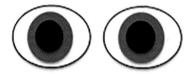

d-i.

Fig. 11.1d-i. Demonstrates normal pupils in the dark.

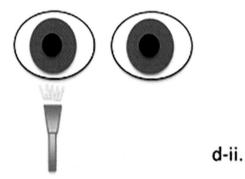

d-ii.

Fig. 11.1d-ii. On direct stimulation of a normal pupil, with a bright, focussed light source, the pupil constricts briskly.

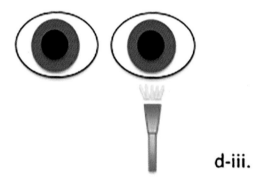

d-iii.

Fig. 11.1d-iii. The torch should be swung rapidly to stimulate the other pupil, which will show mild dilation.

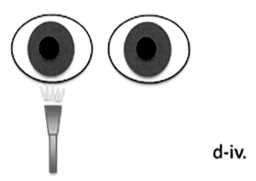

d-iv.

Fig. 11.1d-iv. Swinging the torch back to the normal pupil, will elicit a brisk response.

Light-Near Dissociation (Figs. 11.1e-i and 11.1e-ii)

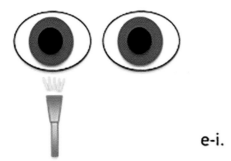

e-i.

Fig. 11.1e-i. Direct light reflex is sluggish.

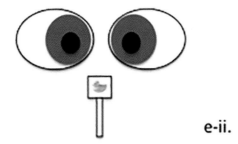

e-ii.

Fig. 11.1e-ii. Using an accommodative target, the subject demonstrates a better "near" response.

Chapter 12

CLINICAL EXAMINATIONS

12.1 Approaches to Visual Acuity

Learning Objectives

• Assessment of visual acuity is the first mandatory step to any ophthalmic evaluation

Flowchart

1. Visual Acuity Checking

Equipment
- Check that correct equipment is available
- Snellen / ETDRS chart
- Occluder and pinhole (Fig. 12.1)

UCVA
- Check and record the patient's uncorrected visual acuity (UCVA)
- People who normally wear glasses must be tested with glasses
- Place patient 3 or 6 metres from chart, depending on chart
- Use adequate illumination
- One eye should be checked each time, while occluding the fellow eye (with occluder or palm of hand)
- Ask patient to read each consecutive line from the top of the chart
- Record the line containing the smallest letters that can be read correctly by the patient

Pinhole
- Place a pinhole over the tested eye, while occluding the fellow eye
- Check and record the patient's visual acuity with pinhole with the same technique as for UCVA testing
- If there is an improvement compared to UCVA, this is indicative of a refractive error

2. Measurements in Patients with Poor Visual Acuity

| If the patient is unable to read the topmost line | ➡ | Walk the patient towards the chart so that he/she is 3 metre away (VA 3/60) | ➡ | Ask patient to count fingers at 1 metre. |

⬇

| Check for perception of light in a dim room | ⬅ | Check if patient can appreciate hand movements. | ⬅ | Ask patient to count fingers close to face |

⬇

No perception of light

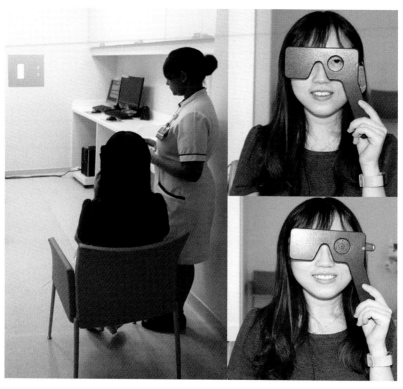

Fig. 12.1. The picture on left shows the proper set up for visual acuity measurement. The pictures on right show the proper way of holding the occluder without pinhole first (top-right) and then with pinhole (bottom-right) while checking visual acuity for left eye.

Take home messages

• Make sure the patents sits at a correct distance.

• Patient's other eye must be occluded properly.

12.2 Cover Test

Learning Objectives
To evaluate a patient presenting with / suspected to have an ocular deviation.

Pre-requisites for Cover Test
- Eye movement capability
- Image formation and perception
- Foveal fixation in each eye
- Attention and cooperation

3 Types of Cover Test
- Cover-uncover test (steps of this will be covered here only)
  - Detects presence of manifest strabismus
  - Differentiates heterophoria from heterotropia
- Alternate cover test (with or without prisms)
  - Measures total deviation, regardless of whether it is latent or manifest
  - Does not specify how much of each type of deviation is present
- Simultaneous prism cover test
  - Determines actual heterotropia when both eyes are uncovered
  - Performed by covering the fixating eye at the same time the prism is placed in front of the deviating eye, using increasing prism powers until the deviated eye no longer shifts

Cover tests should be performed with fixation at distance and at near, with and without glasses (if present).

Cover-Uncover Test

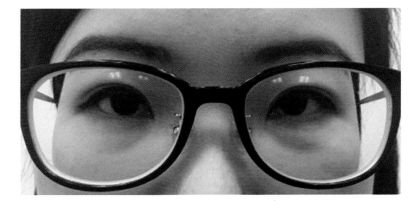

Fig. 12.2. Fixating on a distant / near target.

1. Inspect (Fig. 12.2)
   - Ask patient to fixate on a distant (or near) target
   - Look for any glasses present
     i. Can provide clues to type of refractive error (myopia or hyperopia) and type of deviation (hyperopia associated with esotropia)
   - Look for any abnormal head posture (AHP), tilt, ptosis, ocular deviation
     ii. Can provide clues to the underlying condition e.g. ptosis could suggest III nerve palsy, Horner's syndrome
   - If ocular deviation present, confirm with Hirschberg corneal light reflex

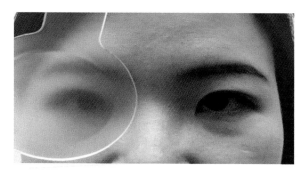

Fig. 12.3. Cover test — on covering the right eye, comment on deviation of the uncovered eye as well as the eye underneath the cover.

2. Cover fixating eye first (Fig. 12.3)
   - Comment on deviation of uncovered eye (if there is movement or if it maintains/ takes up fixation)
   - Comment on the eye underneath the cover
     i. Any dissociated vertical deviation (DVD)
     ii. Any latent nystagmus

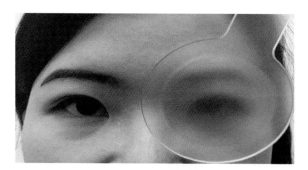

Fig. 12.4. Cover test on the other eye.

3. Cover other eye now (Fig. 12.4)
   Comment on both uncovered and covered eye (as per step 2 above)

Take home messages

A meticulously performed cover test differentiates different types of ocular deviation.

12.3 Normal Fundus Examination

Learning Objectives
- Understanding the normal fundus examination.
- Recognise key structures in the fundus.

Tools for Fundus Examination

The examination of the fundus can be done in various ways. Options include the direct ophthalmoscope, slit lamp with condensing lenses, binocular indirect ophthalmoscope (BIO), fundus cameras, etc.

The main differences between the different devices are the field of view as well as magnification of the image received. The handheld direct fundoscope has the smallest field of view amongst all the options mentioned

Method of Examination

With the direct ophthalmoscope, the examiner is presented with a small field of view. A systematic examination must be done to examine the optic disc, vessels and macula

General tips
- Examine the patient in a darkened room

Red reflex
- Ask patient to look at light of fundoscope to examine the red reflex
- Use the brightest illumination

Fundus examination
- Ask the patient to fixate on a distant target to reduce eye movement
- Reduce the illumination of your direct ophthalmoscope when examining the fundus so as to improve patient comfort and allow better fixation/reduced eye movements
- Go as close to the patient's eye as possible to get a wider field of view

Components of Direct Fundoscope
- Lens wheel (Fig. 12.5)
- Filter selection (Fig. 12.6)
- Aperture selection (Fig. 12.7)

Lens Wheel

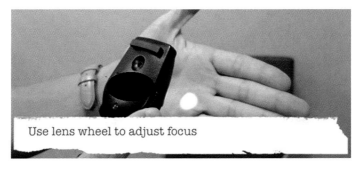

Use lens wheel to adjust focus

Fig. 12.5

Filter Selection

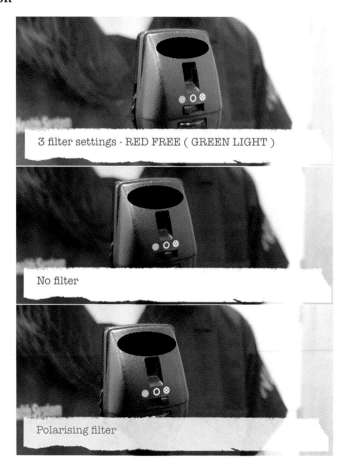

Fig. 12.6

Aperture Selection

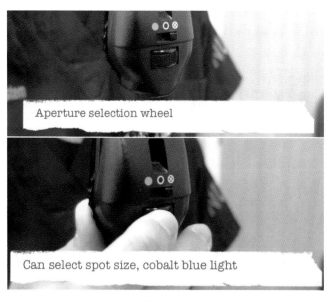

Fig. 12.7

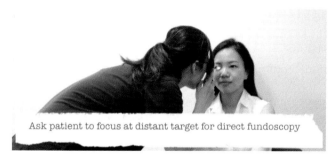

Ask patient to focus at distant target for direct fundoscopy

Fig. 12.8

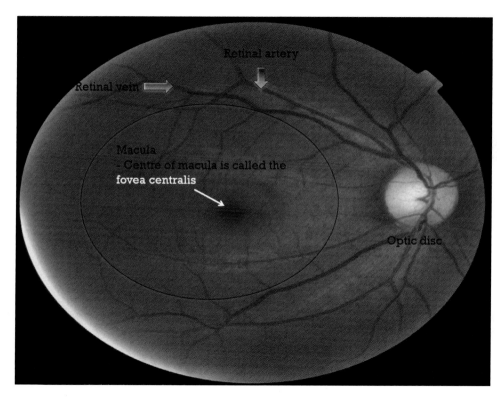

Fig. 12.9. Overview of anatomical structures in the retina.

Steps in Direct Fundoscopy

- Start with a red reflex to assess for media opacities (usually due to cataract)
- Ask the patient to focus at a distant target (Fig. 12.8)
- Dial lens wheel till clear image of retina obtained
- Examine the optic disc, vessels, peripheral retina and macula (Fig. 12.9)

Take home messages

- It is important to recognize a normal retinal anatomy.
- Examine the macula last as this is very sensitive to light.

12.4 Visual Fields by Confrontation

Learning Objectives
To be able to perform confrontation visual field.

When examining the patient, confrontational visual field testing should be performed and documented. Figure 12.10 demonstrates the method of checking visual fields by confrontation. Subsequently, in a patient who is well and co-operative, perimetry (either static or kinetic) should be used to document the visual field defect, which is useful for diagnosis and subsequent management.

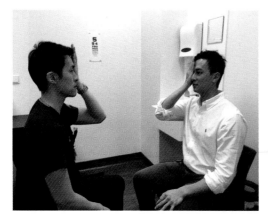

Fig. 12.10A. Both patient and examiner should be at eye level, and each eye is tested individually.

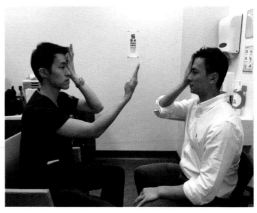

Fig. 12.10B. Start by testing central VF, with fingers placed equidistance between patient and examiner.

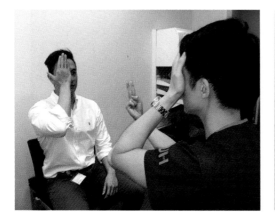

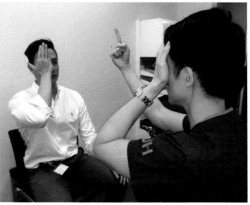

Fig. 12.10C&D. Subsequently, test patient's ability to count fingers in the para-central VF (4 quadrants); with hands placed approximately shoulder width apart.

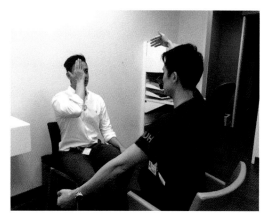

Fig. 12.10E. Check peripheral vision by hand movement.

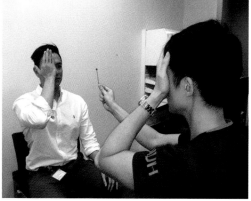

Fig. 12.10F. Delineate VF defect and check for macular involvement with a red hatpin.

Take home messages
- Check one quadrant at a time.
- Check fields in both eyes.
- Check peripheral as well as central visual fields.

References

1. Cover tests. www.aao.org
2. Fred M. Wilson, *et al. Practical Ophthalmology – A Manual for Beginning Residents* , 4th ed..

GLOSSARY

1. AAU: Acute Anterior Uveitis
2. AC: Anterior Chamber
3. ACE: Angiotensin Converting Enzyme
4. AION: Anterior Ischaemic Optic Neuropathy
5. AKC: Atopic Keratoconjunctivitis
6. AMD: Age Related Macular Degeneration
7. ANA: Antinuclear Antibodies
8. ANCA: Anti-neutrophil Cytoplastic Antibodies
9. APAC: Acute Primary Angle Closure
10. AREDS: Age-related Eye Disease
11. AS-OCT: Anterior Segment Optical Cohorence Tomogaphy
12. BCC: Basal Cell Carcinoma
13. BCNS: Basal Cell Nevus Syndrome
14. BCVA: Best-corrected Visual Acuity
15. BIO: Binocular Indirect Ophthalmoscope
16. BRAO: Branch Retinal Artery Occlusion
17. BRVO: Branch Retinal Vein Occlusion
18. CACG: Chronic Angle Closure Glaucoma
19. CB: Ciliary Body
20. CCF: Carotico-cavernous Fistual
21. CME: Cystoid Macular Oedema
22. CMV: Cytomegalo Virus
23. CN: Cranial Nerve
24. CNVM: Choroidal Neovascular Membrane
25. CPEO: Chronic Progressive External Ophthalmoplegia
26. CRAO: Central Retinal Artery Occlusion
27. CRVO: Central Retinal Vein Occlusion
28. CSCR: Central Serous Choroidoretinopathy
29. CSF: Cerebrospinal Fluid

30. CSME: Clinically Significant Macular Oedema
31. CT: Computer Tomography
32. DCR: Dacryocystorhinostomy
33. DM: Diabetes Mellitus
34. DRP: Diabetic Retinopathy Photograph
35. DVD: Dissiciated Vertical Deviation
36. ECCE: Extracapsular Cataract Extraction
37. ELDR: Endoscopic Lacrimal Ductal Recanalization
38. ESR: Erythrocyte Sedimentation Rate
39. ETDRS: Early Treatment Diabetic Retinopathy Study
40. EUA: Examination Under Anaesthesia
41. FB: Foreign Body
42. FBC: Full Blood Count
43. FDDT: Fluorescein Dye Disappearance Test
44. FEVR: Familial Exudative Vitreoretinopathy
45. FFA: Fundus Fluorescin Angiogram
46. FPL: Forced Preferential Looking
47. GHT: Glaucoma Hemifield Test
48. GO: Grave's Orbitopathy
49. GPA: Glaucoma Progression Analysis
50. GPC: Giant Papillary Conjunctivitis
51. HAART: Highly Active Antiretoviral Therapy
52. HIV: Human Immunodeficiency Virus
53. HLA: Human Leucocytic Antigen
54. HM: Hand Movement
55. HRT: Heidelberg Retinal Tomography
56. HSV: Herpes Simplex Virus
57. HTN: Hypertention
58. HZO: Herpes Zoster Ophthalmicus
59. HZV: Herpes Zoster Virus
60. ICCE: Intracapsular Cataract Extraction
61. ICE Syndrome: Irido-corneal-endothelial Syndrome
62. ICG: Indocyanin Green
63. ICP: Intracranial Pressure
64. IIH: Idiopathic Intracranial Hypertension
65. IOL: Intraocular Lens
66. ION: Ischemic Optic Neuropathy
67. IOP: Intraocular Pressure
68. IRMA: Intraretinal Microvascular Anomaly
69. IRU: Immune Reconstitution Uveitis

70. IVDU: Intravenous Drug Users
71. JIA: Juvenile Idiopathic Arthritis
72. JRA: Juvenile Rheumatoid Arthritis
73. KPs: Keratic Precipitates
74. LPS: Levator Palpabrae Superioris
75. MD: Mean Deviation
76. MG: Myasthenia Gravis
77. MRD: Margin-reflex Distance
78. MRI: Magenic Resonance Imaging
79. MRSA: Methicillin Resistant Staphylococcus Aureus
80. MSS: Moh's Micrographic Surgery
81. NAAION:Non-arteritic Anterior Ischaemic Optic Neuropathy
82. NLDO: Nasolacrimal Duct Obstruction
83. NMO: Neuromyelitis Optica (NMO)
84. NMOSD: NMO Spectrum Disorder
85. NPDR: Non-proliferative Diabetic Retinopathy
86. NSAID: Non-steroidal Anti-inflammatory Drugs
87. NVA: Neovascularisation of the Angle
88. NVD: Neovascular Disc
89. NVE: Neovascular Elsewhere
90. NVG: Neovascular Glaucoma
91. OCP: Ocular Cicatricial Pemphigoid
92. OCT: Optical Cohorence Tomogaphy
93. OKN: Optokinetic Nystagmus
94. OSNM: Optic Nerve Sheath Meningioma
95. PAC: Primary Angle Closure
96. PACG: Primary Angle Closure Glaucoma
97. PAS: Peripheral Anterior Synechia
98. PCR: Polymerase Chain Reaction
99. PDR: Proliferative Diabetic Retinopathy
100. PDT: Photodynamic Therapy
101. PFV: Persistent Foetal Vasculature
102. PNET: Primitive Neuroectodermal Tumour
103. POAG: Primary Open Angle Glaucoma
104. PORT: Punctate Outer Retinal Toxoplasmosis
105. PRP: Panretinal Photocoagulation
106. PSD: Pattern Standard Deviation
107. PTC: Pseudotumour Cerebri
108. PXF: Pseudoexfoliation Syndrome
109. RF: Rheumatoid Facto

110. RAPD: Relative Affrent Pupillary Defect
111. RB: Retinoblastoma
112. RD: Retinal Detachment
113. RF: Rheumatoid Factor
114. RFNL: Retinal Nerve Fiber Layer
115. ROP: Retinopathy of Prematurity
116. RP: Retinitis Pigmentosa
117. RPE: Retinal Pigment Epithelium
118. SCC: Squamous Cell Carcinoma
119. SGC: Sebaceous Gland Carcinom
120. SINS: Surgically-induced Necrotising Scleritis
121. SITA: Swedish Interactive Thresold Algorithm
122. SJS: Stevens Johnson Syndrome
123. SO: Silicone Oil
124. SOF : Superior Orbtal Fissure
125. SUN: Standardisation of Uveitis Nomenclature
126. TB: Tuberculosis
127. TCP: Transscleral Cytophotocoagulation
128. TED: Thyroid Eye Disease
129. TM: Trabecular Meshwork
130. TORCH: Toxoplasma, Rubella, CMV, Herpes
131. TRD: Tractional Retinal Detachment
132. UBM: Ultrasound Bio-microscopy
133. UCVA: Uncorrected Visual Acuity
134. VCC: Variable Corneal Compensator
135. VEGF: Vascular Endothelial Growth Factor
136. VF: Visual Fields
137. VFI: Visual Field Index
138. VKC: Vernal Keratoconjunctivitis
139. VKH: Vogt-Koyanagi-Harada
140. YAG: Yttrium Aluminum Garnet

INDEX

C

D

E